The FAMILY NATURAL REMEDIES Guide

BY
KATHERINE L. TARR
AND
KENNETH R. TARR

Copyright © 2002 by Wendell W. Whitman Company
302 E. Winona Ave., Warsaw, IN 46580

WHITMAN
PUBLICATIONS

ISBN 1-885653-19-0 (paperback)
ISBN 1-885653-83-2 (CD-ROM)
Library of Congress Control Number: 2002113876

Printed in the United States of America.

Cover design and illustration by Jason E. Souther.

Note to reader: This book is offered for informational purposes only and should not be construed as medical advice. For medical problems, always seek the help of a qualified health professional.

Table of Contents

Introduction... 5

Part 1: Life Choices.. 7
   Natural Diet... 7
   Pure Water 10
   Oxygen... 14
   Chemicals in Foods and Household Products 17
   The Truth About Microwave Cooking........................... 21
   Irradiated Food 23
   Genetically Engineered Foods 24
   Immunizations... 26
   Exercise.. 32
   Beyond Physical Healing... 34

Part 2: Home Remedies A to Z.. 39
   Acne 39
   Aging 40
   AIDS 41
   Allergies.. 42
   Anemia... 43
   Arthritis 44
   Asthma 45
   Attention Deficit Disorder (ADD) and
      Attention Deficit Hyperactive Disorder (ADHD) 47
   Athlete's Foot and Toenail Fungus.............................. 51
   Autism.. 51
   Bad Breath.. 52
   Bladder Infection 52
   Boils 54
   Brain Support.. 54
   Breast Care 56
   Bronchitis 58
   Bumps, Bruises, and Sprains...................................... 59
   Burns 59
   Cancer.. 60
   Candidiasis.. 63
   Carpal Tunnel Syndrome 64
   Cold Sores.. 64
   Colds.. 65
   Colon Cleanse 66
   Constipation 67
   Crohn's Disease and Ulcerative Colitis......................... 68
   Depression.. 69
   Diabetes 71
   Diarrhea 73
   Diverticulosis... 74
   Earaches... 75
   Eye Problems 76
   Fatigue.. 77
   Fever 79
   Fibroids and Endometriosis.. 79
   Fibromyalgia 80
   Gallbladder... 81

Gout 82
Hair... 83
Headaches 83
Heart... 84
Hemorrhoids....................................... 88
Hepatitis and Liver Problems 88
Herpes.. 89
Hives.. 90
Hormone Imbalance and PMS 91
Hypoglycemia 92
Impotence 92
Incontinence 94
Indigestion and Flatulence 94
Infertility.. 96
Influenza 96
Insect Bites and Stings 97
Insomnia 98
Menopause... 99
Metal Toxicity.................................... 100
Multiple Sclerosis............................... 101
Nausea... 102
Obesity... 102
Osteoporosis....................................... 104
Parasites 105
Parkinson's Disease and Nerve Neuropathy 106
Pneumonia 107
Prostate... 107
Sciatica 108
Shingles.. 109
Sinusitis.. 109
Skin Problems 110
Sore Throat 110
Thyroid... 111
Tinnitus.. 111
Tooth Decay and Gum Problems.......... 112
Ulcers... 113
Varicose Veins 114
Warts.. 115

Appendix 1: Natural & Herbal Recipes.............. 117
Ear Wax Softener................................ 117
Essiac Herbal Formula 117
Lemon/Olive Oil Drink........................ 117
Liquid Clay 118
Miracle Oil 118
Natural Insect Repellant...................... 118
People Paste....................................... 119
Raw Tahini Treats 119
Shara's Mouth Wash 120
Sore Throat Juice 120

Appendix 2: Resources............................ 121
Web Sites 121
Books and Tapes................................. 121

Index... 125

INTRODUCTION

I have always had a strong desire to solve the health problems of my family without pharmaceutical drugs or doctors. When my children were small, I solved a lot of problems by giving them lots of vitamin C and using garlic oil for earaches. When I suspected that my second child, Rachel, had a hearing problem, I took her to a doctor who told me that her adenoids should be removed. However, after searching a number of health books, I decided she needed vitamin A and E. It did not take long for my treatment to solve the problem. I have always been grateful to my mother who, against the instructions of her doctor, said no when he wanted to remove my tonsils.

When I went to the hospital to give birth, I was disappointed by the way the doctors and nurses interfered with the natural process of birthing. After my fourth child was born, I decided that there had to be a better way or I would not have any more children. I went on to have four more babies at home. That experience was so wonderful that I made up my mind to train to be a lay midwife in order to help as many women as I could to have happy, healthy home births.

Most importantly, in the course of caring for these women I have observed that there is a direct relationship between the health of the mothers and that of their babies. The better the women eat and care for themselves, the more healthy, happy, and intelligent their babies are.

About ten years ago, when my children were nearly grown, I started a health food store and learned a great deal by helping others. In this book I offer you those insights and experiences. At the same time, I learned much from my customers. In fact, it is from them that I first discovered many of the remedies described in this book. The truly special experiences occur when a customer returns to the store full of excitement and tells me that the remedy I suggested improved or solved his or her difficult health problem.

It usually takes great resolution and courage to change your way of living and eating, but the incredible rewards which await you will soon make it all worth while. It is my hope and prayer that the instructions and suggestions in this book will encourage you to take positive action today to become more healthy, both physically, mentally, and emotionally. That is the purpose of this book.

Please note that the book is not intended to suggest particular treatments to solve specific health conditions of individuals. For that, you should consult your doctor.

There is a question/answer board at www.kathysherbshop.com where you can ask health questions or respond to other individuals' questions. If you have questions or comments you can reach me via email at Kathy@kathysherbshop.com or www.kathysherbshop.com.

PART 1: LIFE CHOICES

Natural Diet

No matter how many supplements you may take, your diet is still the most important defense against sickness, aging, and lack of energy. If you do not give your body all the nutrients it needs to function optimally, sooner or later body organs will start to break down, energy will diminish, and you will become a sick, old—physiologically if not chronologically—man or woman. The problem is, there are so many of us who wait until our health begins to decline to learn what we should or should not eat in order to remain healthy. I have noticed an alarming trend; people are developing a greater number of disorders and diseases at younger ages than ever before. Today, even children frequently acquire serious problems which children seldom had in the past, such as asthma, allergies, chronic ear infections, and even diabetes.

Our bodies have the remarkable ability to heal themselves if we just give them the nutrients they need. In our society, not only are we assaulted by polluted air and water, but also by pesticides and chemicals which typically contaminate our food. Also, most of us are deficient in various nutrients. As a result, our organs work less efficiently and are, therefore, less able to resist disease.

However, the great news is that we can change this and allow our bodies to repair themselves by supplying them with the proper nutrients in forms which are easily absorbed.

One important way to maintain health and to gain energy is to increase the amount of raw food in the diet. From 30% to 85% of the nutrition in foods is destroyed by cooking. That is an average loss of 50%. Why eat anything which does not promote health? Raw foods contain an abundance of oxygen. By contrast, oxygen is destroyed in cooked foods. For instance, cancer cells can only grow where there is not enough oxygen for the cells to be healthy. Give the cells adequate oxygen and the cancer cells die because they cannot live in an oxygen-rich environment. When you consume mostly cooked foods, where the oxygen is destroyed, conditions are set up for disease.

Another reason why we should eat raw foods is that they provide more energy. Not only do raw foods contain all the essential nutrients, but since their digestion requires only 10% of the body's total energy, they are easily assimilated. On the other hand, the body expends up to 65% of its energy simply to digest most cooked and processed foods. The reason for this difference is that raw foods contain natural enzymes. Enzymes are vital because they assist in the digestion and absorption of food; cooking destroys these important enzymes. Enzymes begin to break down at 106 degrees and are ineffective at about 116 degrees. Because of this, you will have to eat greater amounts of cooked food to obtain the nutrients required by the body. This results in excessive calories and unwanted body fat. It is a surprising fact that cooked foods are one of the greatest causes of obesity.

The main complaints I hear from people who change to a raw food diet is that they are always hungry and it makes them extremely tired. This does occur during the first few weeks, because it takes that much time for your body to adjust to lighter, less dense foods. Since your stomach and colon need a great deal more time to digest a meal of cooked foods, you feel full longer. Raw foods digest quickly because they possess all the enzymes needed for digestion. As you eat more and more raw food, the body begins to clean out the toxins which have accumulated, and the elimination of the toxins brings the fatigue you may feel during this period.

As soon as this important process is completed, you will begin to feel better and more energetic than ever before.

There is another problem which sometimes arises when you change to a raw food diet. People who care about you may think you are becoming strange, losing your mind, or that you are in danger of dying from a protein deficiency. The truth is that you will be in good company because more and more people are changing to a vegetarian, vegan, or raw-foods diet. Numerous scientific studies have shown that every person needs about 25 to 35 grams of protein every day, and that most raw foodists receive approximately 50 grams of protein a day. Since cooked protein is 50% unusable to the body, many raw food enthusiasts receive more usable protein than those on the Standard American Diet (which is best described as the SAD diet).

If you decide to change to a raw food diet, you can help your body adjust to the new diet by gradually adding more and more raw foods. I suggest you start by setting a goal as to what percentage of these foods you desire to put into your diet; for example, 80% to 90% of your total diet as raw food. Then for the first few weeks you might eat three raw foods each day. This could be a carrot, 1 or 2 stalks of celery, and an apple. Be sure to choose both fruits and vegetables. At the end of the first period, increase your daily intake to four raw foods. Continue to increase your consumption until you reach the goal you have set. I know that before long you will experience a radical change in your life and you will begin to feel wonderful. I have observed that pregnant women using a minimum of three raw foods every single day have healthier babies and recover more rapidly after childbirth.

Raw almonds, walnuts, pecans, sunflower seeds and brazil nuts are healthy additions to our diets. People sometimes think that because nuts are high in fat, they are not good for them or will make them fat; research has shown that by eating nuts you can improve your cholesterol and triglyceride levels and reduce your risk of heart disease. Nuts contains essential fatty acids (Omega-6 and 9). These fatty acids are vital for normal brain function, nerve transmission, new cell division and energy. Studies have also shown that people can lose weight and live longer when they consistently eat a handful of nuts each day.

If possible, it is better to eat organically grown foods. Organic foods are grown without the use of pesticides, herbicides, synthetic fertilizers and other chemicals that are toxic to the body. They contain three to thirty times more calcium, magnesium, iron, and other nutrients, as commercially grown foods. Most grocery stores can special order organic produce if you ask, or you may find them at your local health food store. Even if you have difficulty obtaining organically grown raw foods during the entire year, do the best you can and soon you will find yourself and your family becoming healthier and visiting the doctor less frequently.

Some people experience flatulence (gas) when they first use raw foods. This is usually caused by eating raw fruits with grain products, or not chewing the food thoroughly enough. You can avoid this by eating fruits alone and drinking fresh juice (carrot, apple, etc.). The nutrients in fresh raw juice enter the blood stream almost immediately. You may also obtain relief if you take 2 to 5 papaya tablets after each meal. As your body adjusts to raw foods, these problems will decrease and probably disappear. A wonderful bonus is that the busy homemaker can prepare most raw food meals very quickly and easily. I call this diet the ultimate fast-food diet because I no longer have to cook. If you wish to know more, you can find many books and internet web sites that have valuable information on raw food diets and many tasty recipes.

Pure Water

City water systems are becoming increasingly polluted by pesticides, herbicides, fertilizers, heavy metals, viruses, bacteria, parasites, and industrial chemicals. A study by the National Resource Defense Council estimated that 900,000 illnesses and 100 deaths each year can be attributed to contaminated water. Other studies show that more than 45 million Americans drink tap water polluted with fecal matter, pesticides, parasites, radiation, bacteria, toxic chemicals, or lead. The impurities in water have been linked to cancer, heart problems, and infertility. Babies, young children, and people with weak immune systems are particularly at risk.

Government officials add chlorine to potable water to kill dangerous microorganisms, but what does chlorine do to the human body? Dr. Joseph Price, author of *Coronaries/Cholesterol/Chlorine*, connects the dramatic increase in heart disease in the United States to the use of chlorine in water supplies. In the animal experiments which Dr. Price conducted, chlorine was linked to the incidence of atherosclerosis in 95% of the animals tested. Free chlorine in our water supply causes fats to form the cholesterol deposits known as plaque. It is this plaque which clogs arteries, resulting in heart attacks and strokes.

Chlorine also has many other unfavorable effects on the body. It destroys vitamin E; it is toxic to beneficial intestinal bacteria; it forms chemical compounds which cause rectal, bladder, and breast cancers; and it increases the incidence of birth defects. Chlorine combines with other chemicals in the water, forming by-products which are poisonous and cancer-causing. It damages enzymes and leads to magnesium deficiencies, which may produce many negative symptoms, including high blood pressure, depression, chemical sensitivity, and even sudden death. It increases the excretion of calcium and phosphorus to such a degree that the body cannot absorb enough of these nutrients. The effect of this is to promote osteoporosis.

Officials add fluoride to drinking water to lower the incidence of cavities in children. However, a great controversy surrounds the practice of obliging the public to ingest this treated water. A number of studies have linked fluoridated water to the increased mortality rate from cancer. Fluoride can cause chromosomal damage by inhibiting or interfering with the ability of DNA to repair itself. It also destroys enzyme function, promotes pathological changes in the kidneys, and may produce cardiac arrhythmia by reducing cellular calcium and magnesium. Other studies have concluded that fluoride can cause IQ deficits, learning disabilities, impaired memory and concentration, lethargy, headaches, depression, and confusion. Frankly, if I had no other choices, I would prefer that my children have bad teeth than impaired brains. However, I know that we have other options.

Dr. Hardy Limeback, a biochemist who is the head of the Department of Preventive Dentistry and President of the

Canadian Association for Dental Research, has been Canada's primary promoter of fluoride. However, Dr. Limeback has had a complete change of mind. In a speech given in April, 1999, to the faculty and students at the Department of Dentistry of the University of Toronto, he apologized for unintentionally misleading his colleagues and students on the subject of fluoride. He declared that fluoride additives are a toxic by-product of the super-phosphate fertilizer industry and are contaminated with cancer-causing agents such as lead, arsenic, and radium. He added that fluoride alters the structure of human bones making them weak and brittle, and that the first symptoms of this deterioration is mottled and brittle teeth. He also noted that "In Canada we are now spending more money treating dental fluorosis than we do treating cavities. That includes my own practice."

Many studies show that people in fluoridated areas have no better dental health than people in places which are not fluoridated. For instance, the cavity rate in Vancouver, Canada, which has never been fluoridated, is lower than that in Toronto, Canada, which has been fluoridated for 36 years. Fluoride has also been linked to decreased fertility rates. A recent study in California of 5,000 women shows that women who drink tap water have twice as many miscarriages and children born with birth defects as those who drink bottled water or have filtering systems on their tap water. Both chlorine and fluoride are also known to impair thyroid function. Drinking fluoridated water doubles the number of hip fractures in both older men and women.

When you drink from a contaminated water supply, the toxic chemicals go directly into your bone marrow, fat tissue, and internal organs. The result is that these dangerous chemicals create an overload which undermines the health of your body. The fact is, these toxins impact adversely every tissue in your body.

It is crucial that our water be pure, because water is an essential part of body functioning. Our bodies are 60-75% water and every body organ needs water to function properly. It regulates body temperature, lubricates the joints, plays a vital role in the proper functioning of the lungs, and is necessary for the creation of energy. As we age, we dehydrate because the thirst mechanism is not as noticeable. When you become older, you need to be more diligent to make sure you drink enough water every day. In the course of an average day, the body loses approximately 2 cups of liquid through normal breathing and about 10 cups through perspiration, urination, and defecation. You can replace some of that from food, but the body needs a minimum of 6 to 8 cups of pure water for optimal functioning. Alcohol, coffee, tea, and soda are all diuretics that cause the body, surprisingly, to lose more water than it contains. As a result, they are dehydrating agents. Dehydration often produces many adverse symptoms, including allergies, asthma, gastritis, migraines, fatigue, cancer, obesity, high blood pressure, senility, learning disorders, and many more. In his book, *Your Body's Many Cries For Water: You Are Not Sick, You Are Thirsty*, F. Batmanghelidj, M.D. notes that the root cause of many diseases is dehydration, and that most body pain is a symptom of dehydration.

If you are drinking sufficient quantities of water and you still have symptoms of dehydration, you may want to consider using a special product which makes the water "wetter" and thus improves its ability to enter the cells of the body. I have tried several of these products, and my favorite is $HydraH_2O$. You mix an ounce of this liquid with a gallon of distilled water, and you drink 2 to 3 glasses daily. $HydraH_2O$ alters the way H_2O molecules bind together, enabling the cells to absorb them more easily. Because of this, the cells can also rid themselves of toxins more effectively. I have never tried a product that worked so quickly and gave me more positive results. The first day I used $HydraH_2O$ I was flushed for about four hours. I assume this was because the cells were eliminating waste products at a rapid rate. I no longer awoke thristy in the middle of the night. I found that I had more energy and slept more soundly. The uncomfortable sensation which I had been feeling in my heart for some time disappeared after about four days on the new water.

Since most of the water we obtain from the public supply is polluted, it is wise to filter and purify the water your family drinks. There are many ways to do this. The British Berkefeld is one of the best water purification systems I have found. It is simple and very economical, because it uses ceramic filters that can be cleaned up to 100 times. The actual cost is 50 cents a month for all the water you need for drinking and cooking. Another advantage of this system is that it is not dependent on water pressure. Water is poured into the top of a stainless steel canister, filtered by gravity through the ceramic filters, and exits through a spigot at the bottom. You can take it with you on camping trips or on vacations, and it filters out more than 99% of the bacteria, plus chlorine, lead, chemicals, etc. The ceramic filters are impregnated with silver so that bacterial growth is inhibited. I suggest you investigate the different systems and choose the one which suits you best. It is also a good idea to add a filter to your bath or shower water. Chemicals are able to penetrate the body easily through the skin, and you can inhale chlorine vapors by normal respiration. A Professor of Water Chemistry at the University of Pittsburgh claims that exposure to vaporized chemicals in the water supply through showering and bathing is 100 times greater than through drinking the water.

Personally, I use distilled water for drinking because I believe that it is the purest water available. It contains no inorganic minerals, which many experts link to gall stones, kidney stones, and arthritis. Hard tap water plugs up our bodies just like it plugs up the pipes and water heaters in our homes, and thus it interferes with normal body functioning. Our bodies are made of *organic* minerals from plant sources and they have a hard time utilizing the *inorganic* minerals in hard water. The good news is that since distilled water also dissolves inorganic minerals, you can cleanse your tissues and circulatory system of these undesirable minerals by drinking distilled water. People with arthritis or kidney stones usually report a great deal of improvement after using distilled water for several months.

Oxygen

Prior to the 1940s, the oxygen concentration of the atmosphere was over 38%. Today it is generally around 18 to 20% in rural areas. In large urban cities, oxygen levels may drop as low as 6%! An oxygen-deprived environment is the ultimate growing bed for cancer and disease-causing anaerobic organisms. Remember all those upset environmentalists who protested about cutting down the rain forests? In the long run, it seems they were right. Those forests provide oxygen for the world, and their progressive destruction is reducing the amount of oxygen we breathe.

Not only are we faced with a reduced supply of atmospheric oxygen, but the air we breathe is also polluted by emissions from factories and automobiles. Because of this, it is becoming a real challenge to provide our bodies with enough oxygen. To offset this as much as possible, and to fill our bodies with oxygen, I believe it is a good idea to take a moment several times each day to breathe deeply. Dr. Andrew Weil has authored a two-tape program entitled *Breathing*, in which he explains how he uses deep-breathing techniques with his patients to overcome many kinds of problems. The tapes present exercises to help you learn to breathe more efficiently. When I first started breathing deeply, I found it very uncomfortable. In fact, it was almost painful. But after a few weeks my lungs expanded and I felt invigorated by the deep-breathing procedures. We are a nation of shallow breathers, and this simple technique alone (breathing deeply) can make a big difference.

Everyone seems to understand that the quality of our outside air is gradually decreasing, but did you know that indoor air pollution has become so critical that it is the number one environmental health problem today? A recent government study states that over 50% of illnesses are caused by the poor quality of indoor air. Since lung disease is the third greatest killer, it is important for us to clean up our personal environments. What creates the poor quality of air which we find in our homes and work places? In the first place, our homes used to receive ventilation naturally from fresh air which entered through leaky windows and doors. But now, in order to reduce our utility bills, we often scrupulously plug every opening where fresh air might enter. In the second place, the average household uses more cleaning chemicals than ever before. To prevent the damage that these chemicals do to our indoor environment, you might consider using natural cleaning products. Any cleaning product which has a strong, pungent odor is probably capable of damaging the quality of the air you breathe.

In a research project designed to create a breathable environment for a NASA lunar habitat, noted scientist, Dr. B. C. Wolverton, discovered that houseplants are the best filters of such common pollutants as ammonia, formaldehyde, and benzene. Hundreds of these poisonous chemicals can be released by furniture, carpets, and building materials, and then be trapped in your homes by closed ventilation systems. This may lead to many respiratory and allergic reactions now known collectively as Sick Building Syndrome. Dr. Wolverton has written a book called *How To Grow Fresh Air*, in which each houseplant is rated for its effectiveness in removing various pollutants. Houseplants remove carbon dioxide from the air and emit oxygen, and, therefore, have a significant role in increasing oxygen and cleaning up pollutants in your home and workplace. My husband wonders why I have so many plants everywhere in our home, but I know he is healthier for it, whether he admits it or not.

Another solution is a home air purifying system. I purchased the Living Air XL-15 unit from Alpine Air that ozonates, ionizes, and filters the air. When the ozone function is on (it comes on automatically), the air in our home soon begins to smell fresh and clean, like outside air does after a rainstorm. Because of the air purifier, it never smells bad in our home anymore. I first read about this purifier in *Prescription for Nutritional Healing* by James Balch, M.D. I love the purifiers and have had one in the store and another in the house for two years. Available also are small personal air purifiers that you can take with you in the car or to work. There are other purifiers on the market also, so if you choose this option, look around and compare.

Since oxygen plays such a critical role in the proper functioning of the immune system, a deficiency of oxygen is probably the single greatest cause of disease. Oxygen is the source of life and the most important source of energy to the cells. Air pollution, chemicals in food and water, lack of exercise, and poor eating habits reduce the amount of oxygen available to body cells. When the cells do not receive enough oxygen, they seek energy from sugar fermentation. This forces them to make substances they would not have to make if they had sufficient oxygen. As a result, the cells become exhausted, lose their natural immunity, and are vulnerable to viral attack. The lack of oxygen in the blood is quite possibly the initial cause of most diseases. Bacteria which induce diarrhea and infections in the kidneys, bladder, colon, and many other body organs are destroyed in the presence of oxygen.

From the information I have just given, it is easy to see that the body requires an abundant supply of oxygen to maintain good health. If you suspect that you have a health problem that may benefit from an increase in oxygen, you might try one or more of my suggestions. It may well promote your rapid recovery and put you on the path to better health.

Another good source of oxygen is stabilized oxygen in liquid form, which is available in several brands. Use 20 to 50 drops of stabilized oxygen in water or juice daily to increase the oxygen content in your blood.

Chemicals in Foods and Household Products

In our day people are exposed to more chemicals in the air, food, and water than any population has ever had to endure in the history of the planet. If you eat food that is packaged, prepared, or frozen, you should be aware of the chemicals which manufacturers add and the dangerous effects these substances have upon your family's health. That is only the beginning. Hundreds of other products, including beauty and cleaning aids, to name only a few, also contain synthetic chemicals which have deleterious effects on the human body. Listed below are a number of these hazardous substances.

ASPARTAME

NutraSweet™ or aspartame (Equal™, Spoonful™) is a dangerous chemical which manufacturers add to carbonated drinks, gum, diet foods, yogurt, candy, frozen desserts, juice, instant tea, over-the-counter medications, and many other foods. If you buy anything in a package, read the label to see if the product contains aspartame.

Researchers have documented 90 different symptoms produced by aspartame. They include headaches, seizures, nausea, weight gain, depression, fatigue, heart problems, insomnia, vision problems, tinnitus, brain tumors, memory loss, and hyperactivity in adult and children. Aspartame is sold in diet products, supposedly to avoid weight gain, yet this chemical causes the consumer to crave sweets and carbohydrates. So what is the result? It is next to impossible to lose weight when you ingest aspartame regularly. Since aspartame was added to numerous products, the number of overweight people has doubled. I have observed that when people stop using goods containing aspartame, they can begin to lose weight.

Aspartame is dangerous for other reasons too. It lowers the threshold for seizures and mood disorders and is very addictive. The risks to infants, children, pregnant women, the elderly, and individuals with chronic health problems are very great. If you are hooked on artificial sweeteners, please overcome this addiction! Even a small amount of aspartame acts as a slow poison.

Monosodium Glutamate or MSG

MSG is a flavor enhancer which is used in most processed, packaged, and frozen foods. Studies show that 30% of the population experience unfavorable symptoms from MSG. The Chinese Restaurant Syndrome is one example of this. MSG can create depression, headaches, stomach pains, dizziness, diarrhea, fatigue, elevated PMS, and pain or burning in the chest. This unsafe substance has been shown to precipitate asthma attacks within twelve hours in some people. Children who experience stomach aches and hyperactivity after eating fast foods are often suffering from MSG toxicity. MSG is a potent nerve toxin and long-term ingestion may contribute to Alzheimer's, Parkinson's as well as nerve cell degenerative diseases.

Caffeine

Caffeine is an addictive compound and a nervous system stimulant. Regular use of caffeine will eventually deplete the adrenal glands. This affects blood sugar regulation and leads to headaches, fatigue, tremors, heart palpitations, and dizziness.

Caffeine is also a dehydrating agent because of its diuretic action on the kidneys. If you normally drink caffeine beverages instead of water, you will lack energy due to dehydration. The frequent ingestion of caffeine also exhausts your heart muscle by overstimulating it. Moreover, caffeine inhibits the production of an important enzyme which has a role in the development of learning and memory. This is, no doubt, one of the reasons why America has so many hyperactive children with learning difficulties.

In 1998, 15 billion cans of soft drinks were sold in the United States. Seventy percent of these drinks contained caffeine. In a study partially funded by the U. S. Public Health Service, it was found that only 2 out of 25 individuals could taste any difference between caffeinated and caffeine-free drinks. It was concluded that the reason caffeine is added to soft drinks is not for taste but to make them mildly addictive. This increases sales.

To make matters worse, the average pH of soft drinks is 3.4 which means they contain an acid strong enough to dissolve teeth and bones. Soft drinks, which contain high levels of phosphorus, lead to an increased elimination of the body's calcium and weakening of bones. The dissolved calcium compounds accumulate in the arteries, veins, skin, and organs. Soft drinks are completely lacking in nutritional value. Not only do they have a high sugar content and high acidity, but they also contain hazardous additives, such as preservatives and colorings. If you stop using soft drinks in order to improve your health, you may expect to feel some of the symptoms of drug withdrawal. That alone should warn you concerning the dangers of such beverages. Caffeine is also added to diet pills so that you might think you feel better while you are losing weight.

HORMONES AND ANTIBIOTICS

In the American cattle industry, the government has approved six hormones for use in animals destined to be consumed by humans. The hormones are added to increase the growth rate of these animals in order to get maximum profit. The meat from the doctored animals has a higher level of estrogen and other hormones which affect human sexuality and reproduction. At the same time, the hormones tend to stimulate cancer in people who eat the meat. These hormones have been implicated in cases where children five or six years old grow breasts and start menstruating. Today many children reach puberty at younger and younger ages. Some experts believe that the added hormones are the reason. They suggest that these hormones may also have an impact on sperm levels in men, which have fallen 50% over the last 50 years. For that reason, more couples have difficulties conceiving than ever before.

Animals in the United States also receive about 30 times the antibiotics that people do. Again, the goal is to make the animals grow faster on less feed so that raisers can improve their bottom line. This practice has added to the growing problem of antibiotic-resistant bacteria. Some of these mutated bacteria can cause human diseases that physicians find very difficult to treat. Each year 60,000 Americans die because their medications were ineffective in combating the new super microbes. This is another good reason to become a vegetarian.

Dioxins

Dioxins are highly toxic by-products of many industrial processes. They are the most toxic substances ever produced by man, and contaminate our air, water, and soil. They are known to cause cancer. In 1999, the World Health Organization held a conference on dioxin in Switzerland and determined that 90% of the dioxins ingested by humans come from meat, fish, and dairy products. Americans get 22 times the maximum exposure that is considered safe. Nursing babies receive from their mothers who eat meat and dairy products 35 to 65 times the safe dosage. Your baby would be much healthier if you were a vegetarian and used organically grown products while you are nursing.

Fragrances

Many chemicals used to make soaps, detergents, perfumes, dryer sheets, kitty litter, hair spray, scent strips for home and car, etc, make things smell good but are respiratory irritants. Fragrances can be triggers for upper respiratory problems and asthma. They have also been linked to occupational asthma. It is hard to know what chemicals you react to, because formulas for fragrances are trade secrets and not listed on the labels. In an article in *The Healthy Home*, one author declared, "As many as 20 to 150 hazardous chemicals in concentrations 10 to 40 times those existing outdoors can be found in the typical American home." It is vital to limit your exposure to chemicals whenever possible so that your liver and other organs do not have to work so hard to keep you alive.

Essential oils and blends make good perfumes because they are extracted from plants and usually do not produce the negative reactions that man-made chemicals produce. Using lemon oil in a plain, biodegradable cleaner makes everything, including the carpet, smell good without irritating the lungs. You can find soaps, shampoos, and other beauty products scented with essential oils or you can make your own. One book that contains many natural recipes for hand cream, toothpowder, bath oil, deodorant, and many other useful products is *Natural Body Basics: Making Your Own Cosmetics* by Dorie Byers.

The Truth About Microwave Cooking

It is unusual to find a home or restaurant without a microwave oven. Because they are so convenient and fast, we do not want to believe there could be anything wrong with them. In my opinion, the manufacturers of microwave ovens avoid telling the public the facts concerning the dangers such devices present to our health. Scientific studies in the former Soviet Union obliged the government to ban the use of microwave ovens in 1976. In his book, *The Body Electric,* Robert O. Becker describes Russian research on the severe health effects of microwave radiation:

> Its [microwave sickness] first signs are low blood pressure and slow pulse. The later and most common manifestations are chronic excitation of the sympathetic nervous system and high blood pressure. This phase also often includes headache, dizziness, eye pain, sleeplessness, irritability, anxiety, stomach pain, nervous tension, inability to concentrate, hair loss, plus an increased incidence of appendicitis, cataracts, reproductive problems, and cancer. The chronic symptoms are eventually succeeded by crisis of adrenal exhaustion and ischemic heart disease (the blockage of coronary arteries and heart attacks). —*The Body Electric*, Robert O. Becker, Quill, New York,1985, p. 314.

The conclusions of the Swiss, Russian, and German scientific studies on microwaves can be summarized as follows:

1. Constantly eating food cooked in a microwave oven can cause permanent brain damage by "shorting out" electrical impulses in the brain (that is, de-polarizing or demagnetizing the brain tissue).
2. The human body cannot metabolize (break down) the unknown by-products created in microwaved food.
3. Male and female hormone production is shut down and/or altered by continually eating microwaved foods.
4. The effects of microwaved food by-products are residual (long term, permanent) within the human body.
5. Minerals, vitamins, and nutrients in all microwaved food are reduced or altered so that the human body gets little or no benefit, or the body absorbs altered compounds that cannot be broken down.
6. The minerals in vegetables can be changed into cancerous free radicals when the vegetables are cooked in microwave ovens.
7. Microwaved foods can cause cancerous stomach and intestinal growths (tumors). This may be one reason for the rapidly increasing rates of colon cancer in America.
8. Continual ingestion of microwaved food often results in immune system deficiencies, because the normal condition of blood serum and the lymph glands is altered.
9. The regular ingestion of microwaved foods can cause memory loss, difficulty in concentrating, emotional instability, and a decrease in intelligence.
10. Microwaved foods may cause cancerous cells to increase in human blood.

You can read the details of these studies on
www.herbalhealer.com/breakingnews.shtml

In 1991, there was a lawsuit in Oklahoma involving a patient who had died from a blood transfusion because the blood had been heated in a microwave oven. Heating or cooking a food in a microwave oven is very convenient, but it has injurious effects upon the substance being microwaved. Doctor Lita Lee of Hawaii reported in the December 1989 issue of *Lancet* (a prominent medical journal) that "microwaving baby formulas converted certain trans-amino acids into their synthetic cis-isomers. Synthetic isomers, whether cis-amino acids or trans-fatty acids, are not biologically active. Further, one of the amino acids, L-proline, was converted to its d-isomer, which is known to be neurotoxic (poisonous to the nervous system) and nephrotoxic (poisonous to the kidneys). It's bad enough that many babies are not nursed but now they are given fake milk (baby formula) made even more toxic via microwaving."

The potential dangers of microwaving foods is another excellent reason to eat your foods as naturally and as raw as possible.

Irradiated Food

Irradiation of food is the process of exposing food to high doses of gamma radiation in order to kill microbes, eggs, larvae, and to extend its shelf life. The amount of radiation used is equivalent to giving one individual up to 330 million chest x-rays, which, of course, would kill him many times over. To perform this procedure, food suppliers utilize radioactive waste products from the nuclear industry. We must ask ourselves one vital question regarding irradiated foods: Are they safe for human consumption?

Over 1,000 studies on the safety of food irradiation have been done, and not one of them concluded that irradiated food is safe. On the contrary, most of the studies report a number of injurious effects from consuming such foods, including mutations, reduced fertility, metabolic disturbances, impaired immune function, and cancer. A recent study done in Germany confirmed that ionizing radiation leads to the formation of new chemicals that can cause serious health problems. One of these chemicals, known as 2-DCB, caused "significant DNA damage" in the colon of rats.

Irradiation damages the viability of vitamins and other nutrients, by some estimates up to 80%, depending on the dose of radiation. Since irradiation also alters the natural enzymes in food, the body has to work harder to digest food. Some animals fed irradiated foods have lower birth weights and growth rates, and develop tumors, kidney damage, impaired immune systems and abnormal blood cells. A study on malnourished Indian children showed that they developed blood chromosome abnormalities as a result of eating irradiated wheat.

Another problem with irradiated food is that the radiation can kill the bacteria but not remove the chemical toxins produced by the bacteria before the food was irradiated. Also, since all the bacteria are not destroyed, those which survive are radiation resistant. Eventually, these stronger bacteria will contaminate our food supply. At this point, science does not know what effects these "super bugs" will have upon public health.

The tragic thing is, food suppliers provide the public with irradiated foods in spite of the fact that scientists have not done long-term studies on the effects of such food in the human body. The longest study lasted only fifteen weeks. Because of this, no one really knows the long-term effects of eating a diet of foods which are normally irradiated, such as meat, chicken, vegetables, fruits, salads, sprouts, and juices. In view of the potential dangers, it is incredible that the FDA has already approved for irradiation most of the food in the typical American diet. Since the labeling of these foods is not mandatory, you will not be able to distinguish which have been treated.

Therefore, to protect your health, look for labels specifying "organic" on the foods you buy, because irradiated products cannot be labeled organic. Talk to your grocer and ask what products have been irradiated. If he does not know, ask him to find out. The cases or boxes the foods come in are usually stamped "irradiated" so the grocer should be able to tell you.

Genetically Engineered Foods

A genetically modified organism (GMO) is a plant, animal, or organism whose DNA has been altered to make a new species. Drug manufacturers use this procedure to produce drugs like insulin and growth hormone. However, there is a growing practice among food suppliers also to genetically alter foods to make them resist disease, last longer, and grow bigger. For instance, scientists injected a tomato plant with the antifreeze gene of a flounder so it would be resistant to freezing and have a longer growing season. It is true that growers have crossbred plants, or altered them genetically, for hundreds of years in order to obtain better plants, but only within the same species. But now, genetic engineers transfer genes between plants, organisms, and animals of any species to create a totally new species.

This technology is exploding. More than 50% of the soybean crop and 35% of the corn crop now grown are GMOs, and over 60% of the processed foods on the market contain GMOs. Moreover, suppliers have received government approval to produce at least 50 different GMO crops. This may sound wonderful to some, but many people question the safety of tampering with the genetic makeup of food products, because no one can know for sure the long-range effects such foods may have in the human body. Putting a living gene from an animal or other organism into a plant is imprecise and uncontrolled. These manipulations can result in mutations that may cause unanticipated side effects. For instance, experts are investigating the illnesses of 44 people who ingested foods which contained a GMO corn called Starlink. Over 300 food products have been recalled that have been contaminated by this corn. This corn was accidently mixed with millions of other bushels of corn and many of the people involved admitted, after the mistake was discovered by a watchdog group, that the food supply would never be rid of the new corn. The scenario becomes even more grim when we realize that these new species can cross pollinate, via wind currents and other carriers, with old varieties many miles away and change their genetic structure too.

Many important questions concerning GMOs still remain unanswered. Will the new GMO crops upset the balance of our ecosystem and endanger wildlife, or even create new species of animals, insects, and bacteria? Since more than half of GMO research focuses on developing plants that can tolerate larger amounts of chemicals (insecticides), will this lead to an increase in the pollution of vital food and water supplies? By tampering with our plants, will scientists inadvertently remove or alter the foods' vitamins and other nutrients that are necessary in human nutrition? What actually happens to cows and other animals which ingest GMO corn and other doctored crops? Will this change or affect the meat and milk that comes from these animals? Will moving genes from one species to another eventually trigger allergic reactions in people? And how can they discover whether or not their allergy is caused by a GMO when the FDA does not require manufacturers to label a food as containing altered genes?

The fact is, GMOs have already caused unexpected problems. One type of GMO bacteria, developed to aid in the production of ethanol, produced residues that made the land infertile. New corn crops planted on this land died after growing three inches tall. In 1989, a GMO form of a food supplement called trypto-phan contained toxic elements which were blamed for 37 deaths, 1,500 permanent disabilities, and 5,000 illnesses in humans. Cows which receive the growth hormone, rBGH, have shorter lives and suffer more diseases than normal. Surprisingly, most of the dairy products available to us now come from these cows. Since the milk from these animals still contain rBGH, what will that hormone do to the people who ingest it?

The shocking truth is that our government does not protect the public from these dangers. In the first place, it has not done any long-term studies to determine effects of GMOs over time. None of the GMO products are labeled so it is difficult for informed people to avoid them. GMOs are found more and more frequently in many foods, especially infant formulas, vegetables, grains, dairy products, canola oil, and most animal products. However, you can find foods with labels which specifically indicate that they do not contain GMOs. Look particularly for the expression, " NON GMO." Many health food manufacturers use only certified non-GMO corn, soybeans, and other products, and they reveal this fact on their labels. Ask your grocer about GMO products and insist he finds out. Ask that they be labeled so you know what you are buying. Since foods which are grown organically cannot contain GMOs, they are safe choices.

Immunizations

The subject of immunizations is very controversial and provokes strong emotions in people. This author is against them. If you research the subject, you can find hundreds of published studies that document the failures and dangers of routine immunizations.

A medical news web site related the experiences of a London doctor who identified 170 cases of autism and bowel disease in children who had just received the MMR (measles, mumps, rubella) vaccine. These children were normal and healthy before being immunized, but quickly declined physically and mentally directly after the immunizations. The vaccines contain thimerial (mercury) and credible testimony has been given by scientists and doctors about the relationship between symptoms of mercury poisoning and the skyrocketing rate of autism now occurring in one out of every 500 children in the United States.

An excellent book entitled *Vaccination and Social Violence and Criminality: The Medical Assault on the American Brain,* by Harris Coulter, PhD, describes children and adults who have been damaged by vaccination but not severely enough to be institutionalized. Coulter calls this condition "post-encephalitis syndrome" and claims that the "sociopathic personality" evident in the patients is linked to their childhood vaccination programs. This, he says, is responsible for the increase in adolescent crime and suicide, and the decline in SAT scores in the United States. He also includes dyslexia and hyperactivity in this syndrome.

Other studies question whether immunizations even protect you from the disease. When the Utah epidemic of measles hit about nine years ago, more immunized children came down with the disease than those non-immunized. This gave Utah health officials an opportunity to scare parents into having their children receive the "new" measles vaccine, because the old one had not been effective. At this time, four of my children, including a sixteen-year-old daughter and a four-year-old grandson in my care, got the measles. They took lots of vitamin C and everyone recovered without incident. My grandson never even slowed down during his "sickness." No one had any side effects from this episode except that they are now truly immune from further measles infections.

Even if your child appears to be fine after an immunization, there can be long term adverse effects. The documented long-term outcomes of immunizations include chronic immunological or neurological disorders such as autism, hyperactivity, attention deficit disorder, and dyslexia. It seems suspicious to me that the incidence of all types of allergies, cancer, and a host of other diseases have exploded since immunizations became routine. Such conditions scarcely existed 30 years ago before the government began its national program in 1977, for the mass vaccination of children. Researchers have also linked immunizations to infantile diabetes, asthma, crib death (SIDS), obesity, seizures, and many others.

Dr. Viera Schribner did a scientific study of SIDS during which she measured the breathing of babies before and after receiving their first immunizations. Episodes of apnea (cessation of breathing) and hypopnea (abnormally shallow breathing) were measured before and after DPT vaccinations. An analysis of computer data clearly showed that the vaccinations caused an extraordinary increase in episodes where breathing stopped completely or nearly ceased. These intermittent attacks continued for months following the vaccinations. Dr. Schribner's research caused her to make the following conclusions:

> I did not find it difficult to conclude that there is no evidence whatsoever that vaccines of any kind are effective in preventing the infectious disease they are supposed to prevent. Further, adverse effects are amply documented and are far more significant to public health than any adverse effects of infectious diseases. Immunizations not only did not prevent any infectious disease, they caused more suffering and more deaths than has any other human activity in the entire history of medical interventions. It will be decades before the mopping-up after the disasters caused by childhood vaccination will be completed.

Dr. Schribner wrote the book entitled *Vaccinations: 100 Years of Orthodox Research,* which is a collection of her exhaustive reviews of medical literature on the subject. It contains all of her SIDS research.

Various researchers have set out to discover whether or not vaccines have any negative effect on white blood cells, the body's primary immune defense system. They have all reached the same conclusion: vaccines can suppress the immune system. If these scientists are right, it means your child may experience more health problems after the immunization, because of injury to his immune system. The incidence of autoimmune diseases increases as immune function is impaired.

When unexplained infant deaths began to occur in Japan after DPT vaccinations were given to children in a national program, the government prohibited the health community from giving the vaccine to children before the age of two. Subsequently, the number of SIDS cases dropped significantly. Japan has the lowest infant mortality rate in the world. Compare that to the United States, which ranks number 25 in infant mortality. One of the reasons we do not hear more about the adverse effects of vaccinations is that organized medicine and government apply great pressure on doctors to *not* report problems. A 1994 national vaccine information survey of 159 doctors' offices in seven states showed that only 28 out of 159 doctors (18%) indicated that they made a report to the government when a child suffered a serious problem after his or her vaccination.

I personally know three children who nearly died from routine vaccinations. One was a five-year-old girl who was required to get her shots before entering kindergarten. The two others were babies. Two out of three of their doctors denied that the vaccines had anything to do with the children's sudden hospitalizations. The five-year-old girl became very sick after immunization and was taken to the hospital. The doctors could not find out what was wrong and told the mother they needed to remove the child's spleen. Fortunately, the mother was wise enough to refuse. She checked her daughter out of the hospital and took her to a homeopathic clinic in Nevada. There they diagnosed the child with diphtheria, caused by the DPT vaccine. They treated the girl with homeopathic medicines, and she made a compete recovery. By the way, she still has her spleen.

My next door neighbor had a baby who came down with respiratory problems the same day he received his routine vaccination. By the next day the breathing was so bad the parents rushed him to the hospital. It took three or four days to stabilize the baby so he could be taken home. The parents asked the doctor, "Could the immunization have caused this?" The doctor denied it, saying that the baby was probably getting sick anyway. Another baby in our neighborhood also was hospitalized within a day of getting her first immunization but she had a doctor who recognized it was a reaction to the shot and told the parents not to give her any more.

The hepatitis B vaccine is now given to babies before they leave the hospital. Children under the age of fourteen are three times more likely to die or suffer grave reactions from the vaccine than to get the disease itself. Recently, France has outlawed giving the hepatitis B vaccine to children due to documented links between the vaccine and neurological illnesses such as multiple sclerosis, asthma, and seizures.

Since the hepatitis B vaccine was developed in 1987, it is fairly new and little is known about its long-term effects. No controlled long-range, large-scale study has ever been done. However, if you study the reports published by the National Vaccine Information Center, you will find an undeniable correlation between the illnesses (central nervous system and liver disease) suffered by thousands of people and the hepatitis B vaccinations they received four days earlier. A total of 24,775 complaints, from July, 1990, through October 31, 1998, report 439 deaths and 9,673 serious reactions involving hospital visits or disablement. You can do your own investigation by going to the web site for the Vaccine Information Center, which is given in the appendix.

Adults, too, are pressured into getting shots for the flu and hepatitis B. The lack of efficacy of the flu vaccine is well illustrated in a Dutch article about a home for elderly people where, in spite of the fact that two-thirds of the occupants had been vaccinated, a severe flu struck 49% of them and 10% of the victims died. In the general Dutch population, 50% of those who had been vaccinated got the flu anyhow, while 48% of the people who had *not* received the vaccine came down with the disease. It seems, therefore, that the vaccinations provided no protection whatsoever. In the countries where the flu vaccine is being administered, complications from the vaccine continue to appear. These complications include the Guillain-Barré syndrome, paralysis, meningitis, multiple sclerosis, respiratory infections, circulatory problems, and many others. It is difficult for me to understand why anyone would be willing to risk incurring one or more of these problems by taking a vaccine whose effectiveness is in serious question.

The effectiveness of animal vaccines is also questionable. Recently our city gave us a citation for having an unlicensed dog. Since the license required a rabies shot, I went to the city council with information packets on rabies shots, toxicity, etc. I told them I was willing to give our sheltie dog homeopathic nosodes, a remedy used by homeopathic veterinarians. They asked me to prove that this remedy was as effective as the rabies shot. After much research, I could not prove the nosodes worked as well because no one can "prove" that the rabies shot itself works. I gave them another information packet on the effects of animal vaccines and statistics on rabies. I also enclosed a letter asking to be exempt from the city ordinance because of my personal beliefs. Apparently, the city council was unable or unwilling to refute my arguments, because I have not heard from them in nearly two years. Meanwhile, our sheltie remains happy and healthy, in spite of the fact that he still has not received the rabies shot.

Homeopathy is a major health approach in Europe and is becoming more popular in the United States. This technique is noted for its success in ridding the body of the toxic effects of vaccines. If you believe that you or your child may have a vaccine-related health problem, it is suggested that you contact a homeopathic physician. The medicines are individually prepared for the particular symptoms the person is experiencing. If you decide you must get an immunization, there are also homeopathic remedies that you can take before and after the immunization in order to obtain protection against the effects of the vaccine. One doctor advises that his patients use, after receiving a vaccine, the homeopathic Thuja 30 C.

A few years ago I had a conversation with a pediatric immunologist. I questioned him somewhat about what he did. He replied that he made vaccines. Since I was curious as to whether or not he immunized his own children, I put the question to him. His answer surprised me, for he declared firmly, "No, never! There's no one who could make me do that to my children! I know what is in the vaccines and would never put them into my children." I had already heard that many of the scientists who make these vaccines refuse to administer them to their own children, but now had some confirmation that the rumors were true.

There are hundreds of doctors and scientists who are raising their voices against the harmful effects of immunizations, but you will not hear much about their protests unless you seek alternative information in books and on the internet. We are fortunate that the internet has made it possible to find vast amounts of information on every kind of subject. While I was doing the research about rabies, I began at www.shirleys-wellness-cafe.com, which has hundreds of links to other sites.

Exercise

Proper physical exercise is just as important as good diet if you want to have a healthy body. However, the sad truth is that, for most Americans, regular exercise is the exception rather than the rule. It is well known that when people do not exercise frequently, their bodies become weak and flabby and prone to many kinds of diseases. We have all heard, and perhaps used ourselves, the typical excuses for not exercising. We are too busy, too tired, too old, or have some physical condition which prevents us from exercising.

However, the truth is that these excuses are nothing but rationalizations. What they actually reveal is that we do not truly understand the vital role exercise has in living long, healthy lives. If we engage in proper daily exercise, we will gain time because we can work more efficiently and accomplish more. In a short time we will sleep better and our bodies will have more energy and vitality, and thus we will not feel nearly as tired. Moreover, the physical impairments some people use as excuses often disappear in the course of our exercise program.

Let me address one type of physical condition that many people use as an excuse not to walk or jog. They say they cannot do aerobic exercises because they have problems with their feet. Often the people who say this are overweight. They do not seem to realize that if they walked a few miles a day, they would be engaging in one of the best exercises to burn calories and to lose the weight which is the culprit putting so much stress on their feet. They could make more rapid progress, of course, if at the same time they tried to eat a healthy diet and reduce their intake of calories. Also, there are many exercises, such as bicycling and swimming, which can make them aerobically fit without applying stress to their feet.

However, if a person with weight problems finds it convenient to walk in order to become fit, all he or she has to do is begin by walking a short distance at a slow rate. This might be no more than a quarter of a mile in 5 or 6 minutes. The important thing at the beginning is not the distance nor the speed, but the fact that she has started and is out there doing her best. Then she can gradually increase the distance and the rate over a period of months. I suggest she give herself the final goal of walking from two to four miles at the rate of 15 to 17 minutes per mile. This should be done 4 or 5 times a week. It might take some people a year to reach this goal, but they will be proud of themselves when they do, and their fitness and weight will gradually improve as the months pass. Of course, others may be able to progress faster and walk (or jog) longer distances at faster rates.

In one study described in *Fitness After Fifty*, by Heber deVries, more than 200 men and women (ages 56 to 87) participated in a fitness program. The program combined a walk-jog routine, calisthenics, and stretching. The sessions lasted one hour and were done three to five times a week (at least every other day). After six weeks of exercises, the participants began to see changes. Their blood pressure readings dropped, their percentage of bad body fat decreased, their oxygen capacity increased, and their muscular strength improved. These improvements continued until about 42 weeks when they reached peak levels of fitness. They reported sleeping better, less joint pain, and they no longer experienced constipation. The men and women 60 to 70 years old became as fit and energetic as those 20 to 30 years younger. The truth is, proper exercise reduces your chronological age.

The interesting thing about the study mentioned above is that the exercises these older people did were not at all stressful, painful, or strenuous. *Fitness After Fifty* is an excellent guide to physical fitness and I recommend it for older people and even those who are young. Younger people may desire, of course, to increase the length and difficulty of the exercises.

In recent decades health scientists and exercise therapists have proven that exercise increases the strength and efficiency of the heart muscles, increases oxygen in the blood stream by improving lung capacity, stops mineral loss from bones, delays aging, increases energy, and helps prevent depression and anxiety.

The minimum time to exercise for good results is 20 minutes at least 4 or 5 times a week. This should be increased to at least 30 minutes as you get stronger. Walking briskly, slow jogging, swimming, bicycling, and jumping on a trampoline are all good exercises. My husband walks two and a half miles on the local high school track, four or five times a week, at the rate of at least sixteen minutes a mile. The other three days of the week, he uses an exercycle for 20 minutes and does several muscle-building calisthenics. As for me, I love the trampoline. In warm weather I use the big one outside and in cold weather the little on in the house. I usually put on music and a timer to make sure I get at least 20 minutes of exercise. Afterward I do some stretching exercises called the five rites. These are ancient Tibetan exercises which are said to restore youthful health and vitality. You can read about these in *Ancient Secret Of The Fountain Of Youth* by Peter Kelder.

Beyond Physical Healing

In his much quoted little book, *As a Man Thinketh,* James Allen shows that a person's life is a creation of his own thoughts. Allen declares, "Man is literally what he thinks, his character being the sum of all his thoughts. Every thought-seed sown or allowed to fall into the mind and to take root there, produces its own, blossoming sooner or later into act and bearing its own fruitage of opportunity and circumstance. Good thoughts bear good fruit, bad thoughts bad fruit."

It is the law of the harvest that everything produces after its own kind, which is the law of cause and effect. The Bible states this principle in several ways. Proverbs 23:7 declares, "For as he [a man] thinketh in his heart, so is he." In Galatians 6:7 the apostle Paul says, "For whatsoever a man soweth, that shall he also reap." Everything we send out will return to us abundantly. Even our thoughts go out as a magnetic energy to gather more of what we are creating unto ourselves.

That means we are creators. We create with our thoughts, emotions, words, and actions. And whatever we create, we receive more of the same in return. Strong emotions are the fuel that powers our creations. We participate in creation whether we intend to or not. In other words, we create consciously or subconsciously. Most of us are subconscious creators who do not want to take responsibility for what we create. Negative emotions such as hate, fear, anger, and guilt will bring into your life more of the same. If you think the world is a horrible place, you will automatically draw all kinds of things into your life to prove how bad the world is, and that will be *your* creation and *your* truth. If you do not love yourself, you will draw into your life people who will not show you love or respect.

Researchers estimate that the average person has 50,000 thoughts every day, and that 95% of them are in some way negative. By choosing a new thought, we automatically replace all the old thoughts. Every moment of every day we can choose what kind of thoughts we wish to have. Our society has programmed criticism and negativity deeply within us, but each time we think of criticizing, we have the power to make a better choice: appreciation instead of criticism.

We are all created in God's image, and because that is true, He has given us a measure of His creative power through our thoughts and words. We always receive what we create and we are always creating. God makes no restrictions about what we create, but leaves it to the law of cause and effect to teach us how to use His creative powers as well as instruction in His Word. If we do not like what we create, we can begin again. The opportunity to choose again is always before us. The truth is, with God's help, you are the only one who can change your life. You are the only one responsible for your happiness, health, or anything else in your life. The world is in the condition it is because of the choices we have made or have failed to make. God has no responsibility for the world's conditions. Since the Fall of Adam, we collectively have made it this way. God gives us creative power but does not step in and remove the consequences of how we use that power. He does not do for us what we have the power to do for ourselves. If we understand this, we can change many things that harm us and truly have dominion over our lives.

The next time something negative happens to you, you might ask yourself, "What do I want to become in relation to this? Do

I want to add negativity to this situation or practice my godlike attributes? What would love do now?" When God looks upon us, He loves us in spite of our shortcomings. This is an example of how we should see others. See their positive characteristics and what they have the potential to become. Do not look for the bad, or by your thoughts you will make it harder for that person to rise above his current situation. We should remember that each person is truly doing the best he can, based on his current beliefs and thoughts about himself. God loves that person and when you also love that person, you make it a little easier for him to think good about himself, develop his positive attributes, and begin to seek after God.

It is through your thoughts, feelings, and the power of God that you have the power to change your life. Prayer, meditation, and quieting the mind are the mental processes which change your ideas and emotions, and thus your life. When a thought comes into your mind that will not bring the results you desire, cancel it immediately and replace it with an affirmation. Negative emotions and thoughts continuously drain energy, while positive emotions and thoughts energize you with peace, love, and happiness. Replacing negative actions and ideas redirects your energy toward creativity and happiness. When your heart and mind can agree with your affirmation, it will produce results beyond your expectations. The great value of affirmations, in contrast to pleading prayers, is that they transform what needs changing—your mind (attitudes) and your heart (beliefs). In other words, the changes are easier to attain when you make statements in the affirmative.

Now I will give you examples of positive affirmations. After reading them, I suggest you make up your own, according to your needs. Always word them in the present tense as if the goal has already been achieved. The statement "I will lose weight" is ineffective, because the underlying idea is "I am not doing that now but later I hope to." Instead, say, "I am losing weight and every day I look better and better." I found it helpful to choose the ones I needed and to record them on tape. Then I duplicated them so that there were four sets of affirmations on the tape. I listened to the tape before sleeping and again in the morning before getting up. At first my conscious mind denied, or even ridiculed, many of the affirmations, but I said to myself, "That denial or ridicule is of no consequence. They represent no more than my old thought patterns and are not important." Over time the negative thoughts came less frequently, and finally disappeared. At that point I truly began to believe my affirmations. Now I know that they have helped to improve my life immensely. There are many good books that have been written on this subject, and I have listed my favorites under Resources.

SAMPLE AFFIRMATIONS:

- I have faith that all things work together now for good in my mind, body, and life.

- My body is God's gift to me. I love this gift and I show my gratitude to God by caring for my body.

- Today God helps me with my plan to eat sensibly. I work with my body to nourish it and care for it.

- I deny and rebuke the fear (or whatever) that lingers in my heart and mind. I ask my Heavenly Father to replace this emotion with love.

- I am goodness, mercy, compassion, and understanding.

- I am forgiveness, patience, strength, and courage.

- I manifest divine order around me. God shows me what to do at all times and in all conditions.

- I live in abundance.

- At this moment orderly renewal, adjustment, and restoration take place in my mind, body, and affairs.

- New strength now flows freely to every part of my body.

- I feel good; I feel great; I feel wonderful.

- I watch my words, thoughts, and attitudes. I replace those not in keeping with my new image with spiritual and uplifting ones.

- Since God supplies me with money, I pay my bills in joy and peace, because I know that God now provides me with all the money I need.

- I free myself from all judgment. I am at peace with God and man.

- Whatever the need or problem, God's love is the answer and I am a reflection of that divine love.

- God gives me all power in mind, body, and personal affairs. The power of God now works through me to free me from every negative influence. Nothing can hold me in bondage. All power is mine to control my thoughts, to vitalize my body, to experience success, and to bless others.

Please do not become discouraged. It may take years to change some of your thought patterns. Be happy with a little progress. Be grateful when you recognize the presence of a negative thought. You probably never recognized it before, but now you do. That is real progress. Continue reading books on the subject to remind yourself over and over until it becomes a habit. You will soon see your outer circumstances change for the better as your inner thoughts and feelings become more positive. Some recommended books are in the Appendix.

PART 2:
HOME REMEDIES A TO Z

Acne

Diet is very important in preventing and treating acne. See the section on Natural Diet (page 7). Avoid fried foods, margarine, milk products, shortening, and vegetable oils. Eliminate refined sugars such as those in candy, baked goods, and sodas. Make sure you get 6 to 8 glasses of purified water every day. You can dry up pimples by putting lemon juice or apple cider vinegar on a cotton ball and applying it to the pimples.

One Life Antioxidant Formula: This is the most effective product I have found for acne. It is produced by One Life USA. I have recommended the product to many teenagers and young adults, for moderate to very bad acne, and all have reported good results. One fifteen-year-old girl had acne on her face, shoulders, back, and arms. After one month on the formula, her condition was dramatically improved. The product contains beta-carotene, vitamins E and C, zinc, copper, selenium, manganese, chromium, molybdenum, boron, vanadium, silicon in a base of garlic, and echinacea.

ACK-NEE: This formula by Olympian Labs contains beta-carotene, vitamins E, C, and B6, chromium, and selenium in a base of goldenseal, cucumin extract, and enzyme blend. It works very well for some of my customers.

Zinc: This mineral plays an important role in skin health. Studies have shown that supplementation with zinc helps reduce acne breakouts.

Tea Tree Oil: Tea tree oil has long been used for mild to moderate acne. Apply it directly to the skin or use gels or lotions with tea tree oil in them.

Aging

The older you become, the fewer antioxidants and other crucial nutrients your body produces. Even if you eat a good natural diet, it is hard to obtain optimal nutrition from your diet alone. Therefore, it is essential that you take a good multivitamin/mineral formula to make sure your body gets what it needs. The following is a list of the nutrients people usually lack because of aging:

Glutathione: Glutathione deficiencies are a primary cause of premature aging. Scientists have shown that older people can improve their body's ability to repair itself and protect its DNA by increasing their intake of this amino acid. This retards the aging process. It is important to note that pain killers like acetaminophen deplete the body's production of glutathione.

Alpha Lipoic Acid: This is a powerful antioxidant that is soluble in both water and fat. It helps the body to increase its levels of glutathione and is essential in the production of energy at a cellular level. Take 100 to 200 mg daily.

Antioxidants: By supplying your body with the major antioxidants, vitamins A, E, C, beta-carotene, and selenium, you are taking the most important step toward controlling how long you live and how healthy you are during your lifetime. It has been shown in several massive studies that these nutrients protect you from heart disease and cancer, boost immune function, and increase longevity.

Make sure you get 10,000 IU of vitamin A, 12,000 to 20,000 IU of beta-carotene, 500 to 2,000 mg of Vitamin C, 400 IU to 800 IU of Vitamin E, and 100 to 200 mcg of selenium each day.

Bee Pollen: Bee pollen rejuvenates your body, stimulates organs and glands, enhances vitality, and brings a longer life span. Begin with a small quantity and increase to one teaspoon a day in juice.

Spirulina: This super blue green algae is full of vitamins, minerals, and high-quality protein. It will help bring you a long life. Take 6 capsules or tablets with lunch and dinner, or take a tablespoon of the powder in a drink.

AIDS

Because AIDS is an immune deficiency disease, see the section on Cancer for information on immune boosters. Many of the same supplements are used in the treatment of AIDS. People with AIDS usually do not absorb nutrients well, so a raw food diet with additional enzymes and antioxidants is beneficial. The book, *How To Reverse Immune Dysfunction,* by Mark Konlee, presents a complete program for the treatment of AIDS. Two of the most important parts of this program involve taking the whole lemon/olive oil drink daily, and using castor oil packs on the lower abdomen to increase the patient's count of white blood cells. The lemon/olive oil drink is taken 2 or 3 times a day and returns the body to a more alkaline condition so that it can absorb nutrients. Some claim it even inactivates the HIV virus. See Natural and Herbal Recipes (page 117) for how to make it. If you are pregnant and are HIV positive, be aware that AZT usually causes enlarged craniums and slow development in newborns. In one experiment researchers found that supplementing HIV positive pregnant women with vitamin A reduced the rate of HIV transmission from mother to baby to 8.3% compared to 25.5% of the control group. This was as effective as AZT but did not cause the enlarged cranium and delayed development of the babies.

Alpha Lipoic Acid: Scientists have found that Alpha Lipoic Acid can inhibit replication of HIV-1 and other viruses through its ability to bind directly to DNA. In a recent study of 12 people with AIDS that were given Alpha Lipoic Acid, glutathione levels were increased by 100%, vitamin C levels by 90%, and T4 cells by 66%. At the same time oxidative stress declined in 70% of the participants. Try 100 to 200 mg daily.

Amino Acid Therapy: People with AIDS show a marked imbalance in the amino acid pool of their bodies. They are usually deficient in methionine, cystine, and cysteine, while they have very high levels of arginine and glutamate. This imbalance may be causing some of the symptoms of AIDS. Adding 1,000 mg daily of each of the deficient amino acids could make a difference in how you feel.

Vitamin A: This vitamin plays an essential role in immunity and in the maintenance of the body's mucous membranes. Also, it increases white blood cell count. Take one to two tablespoons of cod liver oil daily, or 25,000 IU of fish liver oil or beta-carotene.

Methylcobalamin: This is the form of vitamin B-12 used by the brain and nervous system. It slows the progression of HIV+ patients to AIDS and helps prevent neurological problems. Place a one-milligram lozenge under your tongue three times a day.

Allergies

Allergies are the immune system's response to a substance that would not normally cause a problem. It makes sense that improving your diet, utilizing pure water and air, and taking immune system builders will enable your body to heal itself and avoid developing allergies. I know this can be done because I had allergies most of my life and I overcame my problems by taking the steps just mentioned. Fortunately, I have not suffered from allergies for about eight years. Please see the section on Asthma because the suggestions given there also work for allergies.

Respir-All: This is a wonderful allergy formula from Now Foods. It is one of the most popular formulas in my store because it has a high success rate. It contains quercetin, nettle extract, bromelain, licorice extract, vitamins C and B-6, magnesium, and zinc.

MSM: This is a natural body sulfur. People with chronic severe allergies have reported substantial or complete relief of symptoms after taking 2,000 to 5,000 mg of MSM daily. MSM supports the development of new cells and cleanses the bloodstream of impurities. It is absorbed better when taken with vitamin C.

Colloidal Silver: This is an effective anti-bacteria/virus agent. Use the kind that looks like water (15-20 parts per million). Put this liquid in a spray bottle and spray it into your eyes when they feel itchy and watery. Allergies often begin in the eyes and mucous membranes, so if you keep your eyes and sinuses clean, you will strengthen your body's ability to minimize symptoms. It works well on my granddaughter who has hay fever.

Magnesium: Use 500 to1,000 mg a day. This is a natural antihistamine which relaxes bronchial muscles during allergic reactions.

Vitamin C: It blocks allergic reactions, builds healthy mucous membranes, and fights inflammation. Take 1,000 mg three times a day in allergy season.

Vitamin A or Beta-carotene: This nutrient is necessary for healthy mucous membranes. You can take it in a multivitamin or use 25,000 IU daily during the allergy season.

Anemia

Deficiency in iron can result in fatigue, itchy skin, and irritability. Ferrous sulfate, which is the most common iron prescribed, is hard to assimilate and causes constipation. To assimilate iron easily, the body requires vitamins C, E, B-12, and adequate levels of HCl (hydrochloric acid). Take iron during meals. At the same time take a tablespoon of apple cider vinegar to help absorb the iron.

Chlorophyll: The next best thing to a blood transfusion is a bottle of liquid chlorophyll. To build blood fast, use 1 ounce (2 tablespoons) of liquid chlorophyll every hour, except when asleep, until you finish the 16-ounce bottle. In extreme cases you may need 2 or 3 bottles. If you have low iron you can take 1 to 2 ounces a day for a month or two.

Iron Complex: This iron formula, made by Now Foods, contains vitamin C, folic acid, B-12, and Ferrochel (a non-constipating iron), in a base of dong quai and red raspberry.

Ferrum Phos. 6X: A number of my customers have told

me that this homeopathic iron worked for them when nothing else did.

Wheat Grass Juice: If you have a way to juice wheat grass or barley grass, you might drink 1 ounce twice a day. It usually increases your level of iron within a week or two. If you are extremely deficient in iron, it may take a month or two to bring it to normal.

Arthritis

According to Dr. F. Batmanghelidj, "Rheumatoid joint pain is a direct signal of local water deficiency of the body. If water intake is consciously and regularly adjusted to the needs of that particular body, in most cases, these pains will gradually disappear." He advises sufferers to drink 8 glasses of water each day. See the Appendix for Batmanghelidj's book.

Glucosamine: In over 300 studies, glucosamine gave better long-term results than anti-inflammatory drugs. Many experts believe that it regenerates cartilage. For best results take 1,000 to 1,500 mg daily. One of my customers had a knee X-ray two years ago and the doctor said he could see no cartilage. She has been taking glucosamine since that time and a recent X-ray showed that her knee now has 25% cartilage. If this continues, she will not have to have the predicted knee replacement surgery.

Chondroitin: This substance helps build cartilage by attracting and holding water. Also, it inhibits the enzymes that break down cartilage. Take 1,200 mg a day with meals.

Shark or Bovine Cartilage: This substance works by blocking the growth of new blood vessels that fuel inflammation in joints. The dosage is 3 to 12 grams a day in divided doses. Experiment to see how much you need.

Bromelain: Since this is one of the safest and best natural anti-inflammatory agents, it can be used on a regular basis. You can take 2,000 to 6,000 mg on an empty stomach.

MSM: This is a biological sulfur that works well for some individuals with joint pain. Inasmuch as it relieves inflammation, it reduces pressure on nerves, increases blood flow, and soothes muscle spasms. Take 2,000 to 5,000 mg with vitamin C for best results.

Essential Fatty Acids: This helps the inflammation. You can use omega-3 in fish oils or in flaxseed oil. Take 1 tablespoon of flaxseed oil daily or 2 capsules of flaxseed or fish oil twice daily.

Spirulina: A group of researchers in Cuba found that one of spirulina's pigments has anti-inflammatory properties similar to non-steroidal anti-inflammatory drugs. In addition to spirulina's anti-inflammatory action, the great nutrition it provides makes it a perfect food for arthritis sufferers. Take 6 grams or more daily; 3 at lunch and 3 at dinner.

Alfalfa: I have several customers who swear alfalfa tablets stop their arthritis pain. They take 12 to 15 tablets daily. Alfalfa contains chlorophyl, vitamins, and minerals which may be responsible for the improvement they feel.

Curcumin: This is a derivative of tumeric, which is used to ease pain and stiffness associated with arthritis. Try 1 or 2 capsules once or twice a day.

Asthma

The incidence of asthma has risen 75% in the general population since 1980. During the same period, the rate of asthma in children rose 160%. Many people believe this rise is related to the increase in the number of immunizations. Also, experts implicate a number of common substances which Americans consume—acetaminophen (Tylenol); certain food additives such as sulfite, used in dried fruits and on vegetables at salad bars; MSG, found in many prepared foods; and sulfur dioxide, employed to preserve foods. Also, sensitivity to certain foods can cause asthma. Milk, milk products, and eggs are the most common. You may need to keep a record of what you eat to see if some of these things trigger attacks.

The steroids which doctors sometime prescribe for asthma can impair your body's immune system and lead to serious health problems. It is best to control the asthma with diet and supplements. A good multi-vitamin/mineral supplement will help destroy free radicals in your body, boost your immune system, and protect you against deficiencies. Certain nutritional supplements reduce asthma attacks in some people. Magnesium and B-12 are very important because they balance the reactivity of the respiratory tract. Children with asthma are commonly deficient in magnesium. Magnesium relieves asthma symptoms by relaxing the smooth muscles of the bronchioles. The usual dose is 500 to 1,000 mg daily.

In asthma and other allergic conditions, the symptoms result from the release of histamine, which constricts the bronchioles of the lungs. The release of this histamine is also the mechanism by which your lungs prevent water loss, so the asthma may indicate dehydration. In one of his newsletters Dr. Julian Whitaker relates the story of an eight-year-old boy who had asthma for more than four years and was on daily medication. Then his mother read Dr. F. Batmanghelidj's book and started giving him eight glasses of water a day with extra salt in his food. In four days the child's symptoms had disappeared to such an extent that the mother eliminated his medications. In one month he was normal. His lung capacity went from 60% of normal on the medication to 120% without medication. Many children and adults drink little or no water and ingest two dehydrating agents instead—soda and coffee. Hydrating your body with ample water is the first step to living free of asthma.

If you use an air purifier in your home, you can drastically cut down on the dust and other pollutants which provoke asthma attacks.

Essential Fatty Acids: These acids are essential. Your body needs them to produce anti-inflammatory prostaglandins. Use omega-3 in fish oils or in flaxseed oils. Use 1 tablespoon of flax oil daily or 1,000 mg of flax or fish oil in capsules twice daily.

Digestive Enzymes: Papaya, bromelain, and quercetin are natural inflammatory supplements that can help.

T-Asthma: This formula by Dial herbs is a liquid that includes lobelia, cayenne, mullein, and comfrey. Lobelia relaxes the air passages so that normal breathing can be restored. The son of one family went from four emergency hospital visits in one year to none the next year by simply taking a dropperful of this tincture at the beginning of an asthma attack.

Miracle Oil: Using 10 to12 drops of this oil in a vaporizer or in boiling water on the stove can make breathing easier by thinning out the thick mucus and opening breathing passages. See the Recipe section to make Miracle Oil (page 118).

Attention Deficit Disorder (ADD) and Attention Deficit Hyperactive Disorder (ADHD)

In the United States more than five million children are treated every year with brain disabling narcotics for this mental disorder. The drug most often prescribed is Ritalin. The problem is, the doctors who write these prescriptions do not tell the parents that Ritalin can cause stunted growth, brain atrophy, decrease in muscle control, loss of self-regard, and depression. According to Dr. Fred A. Baughman, a leading expert and critic of Ritalin, the FDA reported 2,993 adverse reactions to Ritalin from 1990 to 1997. Of these, there were 160 deaths and 567 hospitalizations attributed to the drug. Ritalin is also known to provoke arrhythmia (alteration of heartbeat rhythm), tachycardia (rapid heartbeat), and hypertension (high blood pressure). Research shows that the use of Ritalin is a common factor in the lives of many of the students who have walked into their schools and shot classmates. The drug often produces apathy and violence. When Ritalin first appeared on the market, some parents reported that the substance seemed to help children focus and begin to learn. However, there is good evidence that, over time, the drug builds up in body tissues, resulting in depression and violent mood swings. Many observers are concerned that habitually giving a child drugs to solve problems may also constitute early training for future drug abuse. When Ritalin is no longer given to children who have taken it for some time, they feel lost or even paranoid. Since this leads them to believe that they need a drug to feel good, they may later experiment with illegal drugs to cope with life. I have several customers who were on Ritalin as children and went on to abusing alcohol and illegal drugs to try to find that same feeling as when they were on Ritalin. This confirms to me that using narcotic drugs for children creates adults with additional problems. The cure may be worse than the problem.

A growing number of experts believe that ADD and ADHD is a problem which has been manufactured by the mental health community. They hold that these two "illnesses" are no more than a group of symptoms that have been arbitrarily lumped together and labeled a disorder by the American Psychiatric Association in 1987.

I recommend *The Indigo Children: The New Kids Have Arrived,* by Lee Carroll and Jan Tober. In this informative book the authors present the idea that many of the children born in our day are different from children of the past.

Some of these children are natural-born philosophers who think about the meaning of life and how to save the planet. Others are inherently gifted scientists, inventors, and artists. Many gifted children are thought to be learning disabled. Many gifted children are being destroyed in the public education system. Many gifted children are being labeled ADHD, and their parents are unaware that their children are potentially gifted.

Carroll and Tober estimate that 60% to 70% of the children born today are Indigo. They tell you how to determine if your child is one of these new children and, if so, how you should teach them. Since these children are brilliant, they do not do well in a regimented, repetitive environment. Because they love to think about difficult things and solve challenging problems, they are simply bored to death in traditional schools. Thus, they disrupt classes, refuse to listen, and use their minds for more interesting things. The authors include a useful chapter on diet and supplements. After reading this book one wonders if our society might be guilty of destroying the very children God sent to us to solve the problems of the earth.

The symptoms of ADD and ADHD should be treated as nutritional problems. Feeding your child a natural diet can make a big difference. (See Part 1.) Allergies to certain foods often cause hyperactivity and behavioral problems. A food allergy is indicated if your child has dark circles under his or her eyes. The most common allergy-provoking foods are wheat, milk, eggs, peanuts, chocolate, oranges, sugar, pesticides, chemical additives, and cleaning products. Your child can experience radical mood swings due to eating refined sugar, which causes abrupt changes in blood sugar levels. Eliminate foods high in refined sugar such as soda, ice cream, sugar coated cereal, and candy. Since milk is a common allergen, you can try taking your child off milk and milk products for a month to see if it helps. Robert Cade, MD, a researcher from Florida, and his colleagues have identified a milk protein, casomophin, as the probable cause of ADD and autism.

You should make sure your child receives a good multivitamin/ mineral supplement in order to assure that the child's difficult behavior is not a result of deficiencies in the essential nutrients. A lack of any of the B vitamins can cause mood swings, fear, depression, temper tantrums, inability to concentrate, withdrawal, listlessness, and general fatigue. Doctors at one clinic found that children with behavioral problems had marginal B-vitamin deficiencies. Children who eat a great deal of refined sugar are always deficient in B-vitamins.

Magnesium: This is another nutrient that is almost always deficient in children with behavioral problems. Magnesium is a nerve nutrient and a muscle relaxant. It is also necessary for proper brain function. Magnesium is used up quickly when a person is under stress. The body cannot utilize calcium and other vital nutrients without an adequate supply of magnesium. Some experts believe that you should receive twice as many milligrams of magnesium as you do calcium. It is unfortunate, however, that most supplements reverse the relative amounts of magnesium and calcium. I suggest you give 200 to 600 mg of magnesium citrate or aspartate (the most absorbable kinds) daily.

You can tell whether or not you are giving too much magnesium to your child by his stools. If they are too loose, cut back on the quantity of magnesium. For younger children who cannot swallow capsules or tablets, you can use the homeopathic MAG PHOS form of magnesium, which tastes good and is easily chewed. I have several customers who use this for their children in the evening to get them to settle down for sleep. Also, it seems to help solve the problem of twitching legs and arms in the sleeping child.

Essential Fatty Acids: A deficiency in essential fatty acids is often connected to a child's inability to concentrate. Such acids are found in high concentrations in the brain and are essential for nerve conduction and brain function. Since most Americans lack sufficient essential fatty acids, they may be the missing nutrient in your child's diet. It is a fact that American children get too much of the wrong kind of fat. If you add flaxseed oil or omega- 3 oils from fish to his diet, you may get surprising results. Borage and evening primrose oil are other fine sources of essential fatty acids.

Phosphatidylserine: This is a brain nutrient found in lecithin. Natural nutritional formulas for hyper-active children typically contain this ingredient. It provides protection and structural support to brain cells and also facilitates communication between those cells. It enhances concentration, attention span, and memory. Pedi-active ADD by Nature's Plus and Pedia Calm by Olympian Labs are two excellent products that contain phosphatidylserine and have been successful in the treatment of hyperactive children. They also contain DMAE, a substance discussed next.

DMAE: A hormone produced by the adrenal glands that improves nerve impulse transmission in the brain and helps concentration. Take with antioxidants C, E and selenium. Try 50 mg daily to see if it helps.

Brain Link: This product is a powdered formulation of amino acids, vitamins, and minerals, which the body needs to turn raw materials into neurotransmitters, especially those which affect the areas of the brain dealing with inhibition and planning. The dosage depends on the weight of the child.

Spirulina: Many parents have found that giving their child supplements of blue green algae or spirulina really helps. These substances are green superfoods that are high in vitamins, minerals, high-quality protein, and essential fatty acids. Spirulina also removes mercury from the body. Mercury toxicity has been implicated in ADD. You might want to try 6 to 10 tablets a day or a teaspoon or more of the powder in some juice.

Traditional Flower Remedies: Some people get good results from traditional flower essences from Traditional Flower Remedies™ and Nelson-Bach Flower Remedies. One of their products, Calming Essence™ (TFR) or Rescue Remedy™ (Bach), can be used to relieve your child's stress and hyperactivity. You might give this remedy to him if he becomes agitated at the prospect of taking a test. Some people use impatiens for their overactive child. Clematis can be used to focus attention. The usual dose of these flower remedies is 4 drops in the mouth or in a little juice.

Athlete's Foot and Toenail Fungus

This itching, burning, cracking fungal infection can drive you crazy. Try natural antifungal substances.

GSE Natural Body and Foot Powder: This product contains grapefruit seed extract and tea tree oil. Each morning just sprinkle the powder on your feet and toes, pull up your socks and go on with your life. Within a few days the itching usually stops and the condition disappears. It works well for nail fungus too.

Colloidal Silver: Spray this on your feet each night and let it dry. I have customers who tell me this works very well.

Vinegar: Use up to 1 cup of white vinegar in a gallon of water. Soak your feet for 15 to 20 minutes twice a day for 2 to 4 days. The acid kills the foot fungus.

Household Bleach: Several of my customers said they used bleach to soak their feet in when nothing else worked. Try 1 to 2 cups of laundry bleach in a gallon of water. Soak for 15 minutes. Some indicated they used it only a few times, while others said it took a week or two.

Olive Leaf Extract: Taken internally, this extract has produced great results in healing toenail fungus. It usually requires 3 weeks to 2 months to see results. Use 2 capsules twice a day.

Autism

Autism has increased dramatically in the last ten years. A growing numbers of doctors link this increase to the MMR vaccination. If your child became autistic after a vaccination, I suggest you consult a homeopathic physician to see if an antidote might be useful.

Many parents report dramatic improvement when a natural diet is followed. This would eliminate chemical additives and refined foods from the diet. A good multivitamin/mineral supplement is beneficial, as is extra magnesium and B-6. Some parents have found that using a gluten and casein-free diet helps autism.

The Institute For The Achievement Of Human Potential documents 35 years of success by statistics and case histories. Glenn Doman, the head of this organization, wrote the book *What To*

About Your Brain-Injured Child. The therapy he suggests uses atterning exercises to reprogram circuits in the brain.

In their book called *Son-Rise: The Miracle Continues,* Neil and Samahria Kaufman show how one couple took their autistic eighteen-month-old son, who had an IQ below 30, through a home-based program and cured him of autism. Their story is on www.son-rise.org/history.html. Another organization, Autism Research Institute, is a non-profit group that conducts research and teaches methods of preventing, diagnosing, and treating autism. You can investigate these organizations and read more about how many parents handle autism on the internet at www.shirleys-wellness-cafe.com.

Bad Breath

Bad breath is usually an indication that the levels of normal bacteria in the digestive system are low. When the colon lacks sufficient acidophilus, food rots and produces gas, which rises to the mouth. Sometimes this condition follows the use of antibiotics which kill these "good" bacteria along with the "bad" germs. It is important that you take acidophilus supplements for a month or two after using antibiotics.

Peppermint Oil: Peppermint deodorizes the stomach and the mouth. Take 1 or 2 softgels or a drop of the liquid in the mouth. It also works well for the breath of pets.

Digestive Enzymes: Taking enzymes helps digest your food so that it will not decay and create odors. Take 1 to 2 tablets with each meal.

Bladder Infection

When the urine becomes too concentrated, bladder infections are more common. Be sure to drink 6 to 8 glasses of water every day. Using a tablespoon of apple cider vinegar in water twice a day usually helps by making urine more acidic. Antibiotics given for bladder infections also kill the "good" bacteria (acidophilus and bifidus), which makes it easier for the harmful bacteria, usually Escherichia Coli, to take over again. Recurring infections are the result. You may have to take acidophilus for 4 to 6 weeks to reestablish the friendly colonies so that the harmful ones will not have room to grow. Eliminating chocolate, refined sugar, alcohol, caffeine and carbonated beverages, and using more raw food will help to strengthen the urinary tract. Fresh celery and beet juice is particularly valuable for cleansing and healing.

Cranberry Juice: This keeps the Escherichia Coli bacteria from attaching to the walls of the urinary track so they can be flushed out with the water you drink. You can use unsweetened cranberry juice or concentrated dried juice in capsules or softgels.

Kidney/Bladder: This is an herbal formula from Nature's Way which acts as a diuretic and soothes the bladder. Besides cranberry capsules, this formula is the most popular one in my store for bladder infections. Take 2 capsules two or three times a day with water.

Vitamin C: Take 1,000 mg of vitamin C four or five times daily to acidify your urine and to boost your immune function.

Garlic: This is a natural antibiotic that helps prevent and eliminate bladder infections. Take 1 or 2 capsules or tablets up to 3 times a day.

Colloidal Silver: This liquid acts as an antibiotic to kill the bacteria which causes the infection. One teaspoon twice a day is the dose for adults and 1/4 to 1/2 teaspoon twice a day for children.

Sage Tea: When a number of doctor-prescribed antibiotics failed to cure one of my customer's chronic urinary tract infections, she solved the problem by drinking 5 cups of strong sage tea every day. She uses wild sage, not garden sage. Now she prevents the difficulty from returning by drinking 1 cup a day as a preventive.

D-Mannose: This is a simple fruit sugar which flushes bacteria from the urinary tract. If cranberry juice and acidophilus do not completely solve your problem, you may get better results by adding d-mannose. For bladder infections that occur after sexual relations, take 1/4 teaspoon one hour before and 1/2 teaspoon after intimacy. You can mix it with juice or water. If you experience chronic infections, take 1/2 teaspoon of this substance daily for prevention.

Boils

Boils are inflamed, pus-filled sores that can really hurt. I mix 1/2 to 1 teaspoonful of "People Paste" (see page 119 for the recipe) with water, spread it on the boil, cover it with plastic wrap, and tape it so that it will stay on for 12 to 24 hours. Change the People Paste daily. The herbs in this remedy draw out the pus, act as an antibiotic, and soothe the tissues. Usually the problem is much better after a day or two. Hot compresses three or more times a day help relieve pain and speed the healing.

Another remedy I often use is "Miracle Oil." See page 118 for the recipe. I apply it to the boil two or three times a day. Some of my customers have used tea tree oil several times a day and report that it works well.

Zinc: In Sweden a study was conducted on fifteen people who suffered from boils. The researcher discovered that all of them had low blood serum zinc levels. Zinc is important for any skin problem so supplementation with zinc can speed your recovery from boils and help prevent further outbreaks.

Brain Support

The brain is dependent on the nutrition received through the blood vessels, so the same nutrients which keep the heart and circulation system healthy also support a healthy brain. If the vessels in the brain are plugged with plaque and fatty deposits, nutrients necessary for brain function cannot be delivered. (See page 84 on Heart.)

Many older people do not drink enough water and this may result in brain dysfunction. A 2% drop in body water can cause fuzzy thinking and difficulty focusing on a computer screen or a book. It takes about three weeks of using 6 to 8 glasses water each day to rehydrate the brain.

Vitamin E: This is a potent antioxidant that protects brain tissue. A study of 3,000 people ages 65 and older showed that those with the highest intake of vitamin E (an average of 300 IU daily) experienced the least mental decline over the course of the study.

Silicon: Researchers have established a link between the presence of aluminum in the culinary water supply and Alzheimer's disease. Silicon reduces the accumulation of aluminum in the body. You can obtain silicon in shavegrass and horsetail herbs as a tea, or take it in pill form. Now Foods has a formula called Silica Complex.

Alpha Lipoic Acid: German researchers found that alpha lipoic acid has a positive effect on long term memory in aging mice. Other researchers determined that it protects brain tissues from oxidative damage.

Vitamin B-12: It improves mental function. A deficiency can be mistaken for senility. Try 1 lozenge dissolved under the tongue once or twice a day. The form of B-12 called Methylocobalamin is the one which is active in the brain and central nervous system. Thus, it is better for optimum brain function. Now Foods has this form in their product called Brain B-12.

Glutathione: An amino acid that produces glutathione peroxidase, which is the principle enzyme for controlling free radical damage to the brain. Try 250 mg a day.

Melatonin: Increases glutathione levels to the brain in 30 minutes, which protects the brain from nervous system diseases like Alzheimer's and Parkinson's. Use 1 to 3 mg at night.

Ginkgo Biloba: A study in Australia tested ginkgo on memory and brain function in 48 patients (ages 51 to 79). Half took 40 mg three times daily and the other took a placebo. After 57 days, patients taking the ginkgo showed improved memory skills, while there was little or no improvement in the placebo group.

Lecithin: This is a major source of phosphatidylcholine. Choline has long been recognized as the direct precursor of acetylcholine, the neurotransmitter that is essential for memory. Deficiencies of acetylcholine are commonly associated with Alzheimer's disease and other degenerative conditions that involve memory disturbance and neurological abnormalities. Use 1 or 2 tablespoons of lecithin granules a day in juice or sprinkled on food.

Phosphatidylserine: A number of studies have shown that this nutrient from lecithin improves cognitive function, including concentration and memory. Take 100 to 200 mg daily.

DMAE: Stimulates the production of neurotransmitters.

Start at 40 to 50 mg a day. If that does not improve brain function, try 100 mg daily. Take it with vitamin C, E, and selenium for best results.

Stabilized Oxygen: Patients with Alzheimer's disease improved greatly when they received extra oxygen. There are several goods brands of stabilized oxygen. You can increase the amount of oxygen in your bloodstream by taking 20 drops two or three times a day in water or juice.

Breast Care

Every woman knows that she should examine her breasts for lumps regularly. However, there are also other things women can do to reduce the risk of breast cancer. The best way is to eat a natural food diet with more raw fruits and vegetables.

In his book *Dressed To Kill,* Sidney Ross Singer, a medical anthropologist, reviews a recent study of 4,700 women. The study reported that the women who never wear a bra rarely get breast cancer. On the other hand, women who wear a bra 24 hours a day have the highest chance (125 times the risk) of developing breast cancer. Women who wear a bra for more than 12 hours a day had 21 times the risk as women who wear one fewer than 12 hours. The researchers surmise that a bra tends to block a woman's lymphatic vessels and thus prevents the lymphocytes from destroying abnormal cells. This blockage, over a period of years, causes a build-up of cancer cells, which eventually overwhelm the body's defense mechanisms, and the cancer spreads. The researchers conclude that women should wear a bra less than 12 hours a day and make sure the bra does not constrict the lymphatic system. If they see groves or red lines when they remove their bra, they may run into problems. In addition, women should not wear a bra to bed and should avoid strapless brassieres, those with underwires, and those which push the breasts upward. The latter compress the lymphatic system to a much greater degree than normal.

Several studies have connected breast cancer to the chemicals used in underarm deodorants. The majority of breast cancers occur in the area closest to the armpit. Avoid especially deodorants which contain aluminum and other chemicals. There are natural deodorants that are very effective, so why take the risk?

Other studies indicate that an annual mammogram is not an effective way of preventing breast cancer. It is true that smaller cancers are found, but the mortality rate is the same. By the time a tumor has grown large enough to be detected by an X-ray or a physical examination, it has already been growing several years. Alternative medicine has declared for years that mammograms do more harm than good. Not only does their ionizing radiation mutate cells, but the mechanical pressure of smashing a woman's breast against the X-ray machine can spread cells that are already malignant. One type of breast cancer has increased 200% due to the use of mammography. The problems are further complicated by incorrect diagnoses. In a 1996 study involving 108 radiologists in the United States, 21% of the radiologists missed cancers that had been previously diagnosed, 10% of the women were diagnosed with cancers they did not have, and 42% of the women who had benign lesions were thought to be cancerous. Incorrect diagnoses such as these cause thousands of women to endure unnecessary biopsies every year with the accompanying pain and anxiety. Knowing this, you may want to reconsider taking these yearly tests.

Some researchers suggest that caffeine and other compounds found in coffee, tea, soft drinks, and chocolate can cause breast swelling and tenderness in some women. Try eliminating these things for two or three months and see if the condition improves. It worked for 75% of the women in one study.

Too much salt in the diet leads to fluid retention and can result in breast swelling. You can experiment to see if eliminating most of the salt will solve the problem.

Vitamin E: 400 to 800 units of vitamin E daily will usually ease breast tenderness and soreness.

Flaxseed: This food is a great source of fiber, which is known to help prevent breast cancer. The lignans in whole flaxseed bind to estrogen receptors and impede the cancer-promoting effects of estrogen on breast tissue. Use 1/4 cup of ground seeds daily. You can grind whole flaxseed in your blender and store it in the refrigerator. Put ground flaxseed in a fruit smoothie, sprinkle it on a salad, or mix it in juice or water. Also, you can get flax oil that is high in lignans if you prefer to use the oil.

Evening Primrose Oil: This is an essential fatty acid which is prescribed by many naturopaths for PMS and the breast pain associated with the menstrual cycle. It is largely the presence or lack of essential fatty acids in your body, especially the GLA (gamma-linolenic-acid) found in Evening Primrose Oil, that determines whether you sail through your monthly cycle or suffer from water retention, cramping, irritability, headaches, and tension You probably need one 1,300 mg softgel each day.

Bronchitis

Bronchitis often follows a cold and can lead to serious infections. Sometimes it hurts to breathe and your chest aches.

Vitamin C: Increase your intake of vitamin C to 5,000 mg a day in divided doses. Use liquid or chewable C for children and give them as much as they can handle up to 5,000 mg a day. Adjust the dosage according to your child's weight. Vitamin C works like an antihistamine and stimulates the immune system to fight infection.

Magnesium: This mineral acts as an antihistamine and clears your body's air passages. Use 500 to 1,000 mg depending on whether it is a child or an adult. Epsom salts are magnesium sulfate and can be added to your bath water. Your body will absorb some of the magnesium.

Miracle Oil: If you put 10 to 12 drops of this oil in a vaporizer and leave the machine on all night, the oil will soothe your lungs, making it easier to breathe and reducing your coughing. You can also take the oil by placing 2 or 3 drops of it in a few ounces of juice or water twice a day. See Natural and Herbal Recipes (page 118) on how to make Miracle Oil.

Sore Throat Juice: This is made from cayenne, vinegar, honey, and grapefruit seed extract (see the Natural and Herbal Recipes, page 118). It works well for any kind of coughing or lung inflammation. Sip it slowly throughout the day.

Bumps, Bruises, and Sprains

You can reduce the swelling of bad bruises and sprains by placing an ice pack on the injured area for twenty minutes. A multivitamin/mineral formula which contains vitamins C, A, E, B, calcium, magnesium, and zinc will accelerate healing and tissue repair.

Arnica Ointment: This reduces the pain and swelling of bruises, sore muscles, and sprains. Rub the cream on two or three times a day.

Vitamin C: If you bruise easily, take 1,000 mg of vitamin C every day. This will help increase the strength of your capillaries so that you will not be prone to bruising from little bumps.

Comfrey: Soaking a bruised or sprained body part in comfrey tea can reduce the pain and promote healing. You can also use People Paste. See Natural and Herbal Recipes (page 119) which has comfrey in it for the same purpose.

Miracle Oil: If the skin is not broken, rub a little of these essential oils on a bruise or sprain. It will reduce the swelling and promote healing. See Natural and Herbal Recipes (page 118).

MSM: Use this for joint and tissue repair. It helps with the pain and inflammation. Take 1,000 to 5,000 mg daily in divided doses. MSM is also available in lotions and creams for topical use.

Burns

Immediately immerse the burn in cold water for 15 to 30 minutes to cool the tissues. Apply comfrey ointment. My favorite is Herbal Mender ointment, which contains comfrey extract and ascorbic acid, from Life Research. It promotes the rapid healing of damaged tissues and relieves a lot of the pain. In laboratory tests this ointment killed staph, strep, E.coli, and other disease-causing bacteria in 30 to 60 seconds. One day a friend came to my store and told me that her husband had pulled a pan of flaming grease off the stove, splashing the grease on his leg. He received first degree burns, and the pain was very bad. After trying many things without much success, they used Herbal Mender ointment, which quickly relieved the pain and helped the burn heal faster.

Aloe Vera: Cut open a leaf of this plant and put the slimy, thick gel on the burn. This promotes healing and reduces the pain and swelling. If you do not have an aloe plant, you can use aloe gel in a bottle.

Vitamin E Oil: You can use this by piercing a vitamin E softgel with a pin and squeezing the liquid onto the burn, or you might purchase a bottle of E oil. Vitamin E is an antioxidant which helps preserve oxygen. It also enhances healing and prevents the formation of scar tissue. You can cover the burn lightly with clean gauze.

Cancer

Like most human illnesses, cancer results from a deficiency of vital nutrients. When you supply your body with the proper nutrients, in a useable form, it "knows" how to repair itself. See Natural Diet (page 7). The lemon/olive oil drink in Natural and Herbal Recipes (page 117) can be very beneficial in your program against cancer.

Actually, cancer can only develop in a body whose immune system is not functioning properly. Immunologists say that we all have cancer cells in our bodies, but a healthy body does not develop cancer because its defense system manufactures specialized cells which recognizes cancerous cells and destroys them. The immune system is your body's major line of defense against cancer and infection. The primary goal of *alternative* cancer therapies, which use nutritional and herbal remedies, is to enhance the efficiency of the immune system. The following list of supplements are among those recommended by alternative healers:

Antioxidants: Vitamins A, C, E, beta-carotene, selenium, zinc, the B vitamins, pycnogenol, and grape seed antioxidant work in your body to neutralize free radicals, which are thought to set the molecular and cellular stage for cancer. These antioxidants detoxify cancer-causing chemicals, stimulate the immune response, and maintain healthy oxygen metabolism. Using an antioxidant vitamin formula would be easier than using all these singly.

Essential Fatty Acids: These are necessary for a healthy immune system. You can use fish oil, flax oil, primrose oil, borage oil, black current oil, or a combination. Flaxseed oil helps the body transport vitamin A and possesses antitumor effects. Supplementing your diet with essential fatty acids increases the activity of the immune cells involved in killing viruses and cancer. A dose of 1 to 3 tablespoons daily of the cold-pressed oil is usually suggested. Evening primrose oil is rich in GLA, an essential fatty acid which the body uses to produce the hormone prostaglandin. GLA plays a major role in T-cell function and in regulating the thymus gland.

Magnesium: Studies have shown that a diet deficient in magnesium is related to increased cancer rates, while sufficient magnesium had a preventative effect. Magnesium keeps calcium in solution and allows the body to use it fully. This cuts down on "free" calcium molecules which can feed cancer cells. Magnesium improves the activity of the white blood cells and increases the production of antibodies. A desirable dosage is 600 to 1,000 mg daily in the form of magnesium citrate or aspartate, the most absorbable kinds, in divided doses. The only possible side effect is loose stools because magnesium draws water to the colon.

Coenzyme Q10: This nutrient, CoQ10, functions as an antioxidant, enhances the immune system, slows or stops cancerous growths, and increases the number of killer T-cells. The recommended dosage is 200 to 400 mg daily for persons with cancer and 30 to 100 mg for prevention.

Cell Forte by Enzymatic Therapy: The combination of IP-6 and inositol in Cell Forte has been shown to be an effective antioxidant and boosts the body's immune function. Based on extensive experimental studies in animals and cell cultures, Cell Forte exerts anti-cancer effects against virtually all types of cancers including those of the breast, prostate, lung, skin, and brain, as well as lymphomas and leukemia. What Cell Forte seems to do in the cancer cell is to turn off the switch that tells the cells to divide. You get maximum results by using 2 capsules three times daily.

Beta 1, 3 / 1, 6 Glucan: This is derived from yeast cell walls and activates the immune system by triggering the macrophage cells to attack, engulf, and destroy invaders to the body. This substance activates and mobilizes the entire immune system. Take 2 capsules three times a day.

Ellagic Acid: This substance, found in raspberries, has antioxidant properties and inhibits the growth of cancer cells by stopping cancer cell division. You can use a cup of fresh raspberries every day in season or 5 tablets a day of raspberry seed powder, which contains about 35 mg of ellagic acid. My favorite ellagic acid product is called Razz Tabs. They can be chewed easily for greater assimilation.

Essiac: This is a mixture of four herbs from the Ojibway Indians. The active ingredients in Essiac tea have been used separately in naturopathic medicine for hundreds of years. They purify your blood and nourish individual cells, enhancing their strength and integrity. A Canadian nurse named Rene Cassie used this mixture as a tea to cure thousands of people with incurable cancer. I know four or five customers whose cancer went into remission while using Essiac tea. See Natural and Herbal Recipes (page 117) for instructions on how to make it. The usual dose is 2 ounces of the tea two or three times a day on an empty stomach. You can also buy it in concentrated liquid form or in capsules.

MGN-3: This is a patented extract made from rice bran and Shiitake mushrooms. In Japan, extracts from the Shiitake mushroom are one of the leading prescription treatments for cancer. Breast cancer patients went into complete remission in a seven-month test by taking 12 capsules a day of MGN-3. The extract also produced a complete remission in patients with cancer of the prostate, ovaries, breast, and bone marrow. After two weeks, cancer cells were being destroyed by the patients' own immune systems at the average rate of 240% and it continued to rise for the next six months.

Stabilized Liquid Oxygen: Cancer cells cannot develop in the presence of oxygen, but they thrive in an environment devoid of oxygen. Consuming 50 drops of stabilized oxygen in juice or water two or three times a day puts oxygen in the blood and makes it available for use in all the cells of the body. The product I like is called ION.

Shark Cartilage: This supplement blocks the proliferation of new blood vessels so the cancer cell cannot grow. Also, it stimulates the immune system. Studies show that success rates are in the 25 to 50% range. The amounts needed are large—6 to 10 capsules three times a day.

Skin Answer: This product can safely remove precancerous skin lesions and skin cancer. In one clinical trial in California, Skin Answer was tested on 28 patients. In that group there were 13 keratoses, 12 basal cell carcinomas, and 3 squamous cell carcinomas. A dermatologist treated each of the patients with SkinAnswer cream for 4 to 8 weeks. The patients' lesions were biopsied before and after treatment. With the exception of a single basal cell carcinoma, the cream totally removed all of the keratoses and skin cancers.

Spirulina: Spirulina can protect white blood cells from damage caused by radiation and chemotherapy and improve the patient's recovery time. Use 6 grams or more daily.

Grapefruit Seed Extract: The company which makes this product advances no claims concerning its cancer-curing ability. However, I cleared up three spots of cancer on my face by putting a drop of this liquid on them every day for a month. Each layer turned brown and peeled off until there was nothing but normal skin remaining.

Candidiasis

Follow the diet suggestions in the sectioin on Natural Diet (page 7) and take a good multivitamin/mineral supplement. Also, take acidophilus to reestablish friendly bacteria in the intestine. It is hard to get rid of candida if you are on antibiotics, steroids, or anti-inflammatory drugs. They kill off your good bacteria, allowing the candida to grow uncontrolled.

Grapefruit Seed Extract: This product is a very effective treatment for candidiasis. One doctor reported a success rate of 99% with 297 patients who had yeast or parasitic infections. Use 5 to 10 drops in juice twice a day. For very stubborn cases, take 10 to 12 drops three times a day. It can also be used for vaginal yeast infections by mixing 10 drops in 6 to 8 oz. water. Douche once or twice daily for one week

Olive Leaf Extract: Combined with a healthy diet, olive leaf extract is very effective in destroying candida in the body. Use 2 capsules three times a day of the extract containing 18% oleuropein.

Tea Tree Oil: This helps fight vaginal yeast infections. Use 20 to 30 drops in 2 cups of water for a douche.

Yeast Fighters: This formula by TwinLab contains fiber blend, acidophilus, garlic, caprylic acid, pau d'arco, onion, golden seal, echinacea, and black walnut. Several customers have told me that this worked very well for them. Use as directed.

Carpal Tunnel Syndrome

Carpal tunnel syndrome occurs when tendons in the wrists become inflamed and swell, compressing the median nerve in the wrist and leading to pain, numbness, and limited movement of the thumb and fingers. Avoid caffeine because it constricts blood vessels, reducing blood flow to the hands. Exercise regularly by flexing the wrists up and down and rotating them in both directions. Do this several times a day. You can use a wrist splint if you use your hands a great deal as in computer work.

Vitamin B-6: Several studies show that B-6 can improve the pain and numbness. Many specialists believe that carpal tunnel syndrome involves nerve damage due to a deficiency of B-6, and that higher than normal doses of the vitamin corrects the deficiency. The suggested dosage is 50 to 100 mg of B-6 once or twice a day.

Miracle Oil: One of my customers entered my store one day, wiggled his thumb, and announced, "I cancelled my carpal tunnel surgery!" He had rubbed Miracle Oil on his hands and arms and soon gained full use of them without pain. The treatment did not cure the problem, but regular use of the oil enabled him to work and remain free of pain. I have told other customers about his experience, and many have tried it too. They say it works. See Natural and Herbal Recipes (page 118) for how to make it.

Bromelain: This is an enzyme in pineapple which decreases pain and inflammation. Eat raw pineapple or use the capsules three times a day.

Cold Sores

Cold sores usually appear on or around the lips and sometimes inside the mouth. Outbreaks can be triggered by stress, illness, or allergies. People who get cold sores can usually feel some tingling where the cold sore will soon erupt. That is the time to take action. Before I found l-Lysine, I used to promote healing by dabbing toothpaste on the cold sore every night before retiring. I feel it was the peppermint in the toothpaste that was the active agent.

l-Lysine: This is an essential amino acid which prevents outbreaks and reduces the severity of the cold sore. When I feel that tingle in my lip, I take two 500 mg tablets morning and night, and the cold sore usually does not even appear. If you have frequent cold sores, try supplementing with l-Lysine regularly to prevent outbreaks. There is also an l-Lysine cream for topical use which works well.

Acidophilus: I find that using acidophilus with l-Lysine works even better than the l-Lysine alone. I take 2 capsules of acidophilus morning and night on an empty stomach.

Aloe Vera: Try cutting open a leaf of the plant and rubbing the gel on the tingling spot. Leave it on overnight. Several customers say this works great.

Homeopathic Cold Sore Cream: Some of my customers are totally loyal to this cream. They say it lessens the pain and makes the cold sore go away faster.

Colds

Conventional medicine has made very little progress in the treatment of colds. Many over-the-counter remedies are not very effective and frequently lead to other problems. For example, anti-histamines cause dehydration and improve the growing conditions for viruses. Analgesics may relieve aches and pains and reduce fever, but fever is an important body defense that enables you to fight infection. See Fever (page 79). Studies show that acetaminophen and aspirin can actually increase nasal symptoms and prolong the cold or flu. It makes more sense to give the body nutrients to enhance the immune system so that it can heal itself. When you have a cold, rest as much as you can and use immune-building supplements. Avoid sugar. The white blood cells that destroy cold viruses decrease by at least 50% when you eat sugar, so choose instead fresh vegetable and fruit juices, soup, and other nourishing foods.

Frequent colds suggest an impaired immune system. See Cancer for immune builders (page 60). It is possible that the sufferer's immune system might be damaged because he has been using antibiotics, which have destroyed his body's beneficial intestinal flora. You may have to supplement with acidophilus for a few months to build it up again.

Vitamin C: Increase your intake of vitamin C at the first sign of a cold. It probably will not prevent the cold, but it will help relieve your symptoms and allow you to recover faster. Since vitamin C increases the number and function of your white blood cells, it enhances their ability to fight infection. Take 1,000 mg three or four times a day.

Zinc: Take zinc at the first sign of a cold to reduce the duration of the illness. Your immune system requires zinc to fight viral infections, and if you do not get enough, the cold can last a long time. I like taking zinc in chewable lozenges.

Colostrum: This first milk of a cow contains many immune factors that help fight the cold virus. It comes in capsules and chewable tablets for children. Use 2 to 4 capsules two or three times a day.

Olive Leaf Extract: This is useful for all viral diseases, including the common cold. Take 2 capsules (18% oleuropein) three times daily for a cold or 1 to 2 capsules daily for prevention.

Echinacea: This herb stimulates the immune system and is included in many herbal cold formulas. Take 2 capsules one or two times a day, or use a zinc lozenge which contains echinacea.

Elderberry: Studies show that people taking elderberry extract for colds get well in half the time. You can use the liquid extract or obtain it in lozenges with zinc.

Grapefruit Seed Extract: My favorite formula, Maximum Strength GSE, has vitamin C, echinacea, astragalus, mushroom extracts (immune boosters), ginger root, golden seal, yarrow, and zinc. With this product I can usually recover from any cold or flu within a few hours or in one day.

MSM (Methylsulphonylmethane): This biological sulfur can stop or reduce cold symptoms. Take 2,000 mg twice a day until the cold has been gone for a few days.

Colon Cleanse

If your belly resembles that of a woman nine months pregnant, but you are not pregnant, you need a colon cleanse. Years of eating cooked and refined foods results in a bloated colon. You may have as much as 25 pounds of dried fecal matter compacted in the colon, a condition which decreases your body's ability to absorb nutrients. Intestinal parasites thrive in this old encrusted matter and they produce toxins as part of their life processes. These toxins from parasites and rotting fecal matter are absorbed through the colon walls into the blood stream. In time they can cause cellular alterations which lay the groundwork for many illnesses. Also, the body cannot get rid of toxins and waste products in tissues if the colon is already impacted and enlarged with waste products. This situation eventually inhibits oxygenation mechanisms and the body becomes exhausted. If you are tired all the time, you may need a colon cleanse. The truth is, it is impossible to get well with a polluted colon. However, as soon as the colon is cleansed, other body organs can work better because they now have a place to discard waste products. I recommend Dr. Bernard Jensen's *Guide to Better Bowel Care.* In this book he gives complete instructions for a seven-day colon cleanse. My customers who have completed a cleanse report that they gained energy and experienced improvement in their physical problems and diseases.

An important part of cleansing the colon is to drink plenty of pure water and to consume raw fruits and vegetables and their juices. Raw apple juice is particularly valuable for flushing old matter from the colon. To soften and help remove old encrusted matter, take 1 tablespoon of psyllium husks in 12 ounces of water four times a day.

Clay Liquid: Drink 1 glass a day for three weeks. Clay attracts and binds with up to 40 times its weight in toxins and chemicals. If the clay water constipates you, add an herb like cascara sagrada or an herbal combination (see Constipation listed below).

Flaxseed: Use 1/4 cup of ground flaxseed in juice or sprinkled on food. This creates bulk, cleans the colon, and also supplies essential fatty acids.

Acidophilus: Take this to replace the colon's bad bacteria with beneficial ones which will provide bulk and B vitamins. Take 2 capsules with water on an empty stomach three times a day for a week.

Digestive Enzymes: Taken with meals, these help the body digest and loosen the impacted material in the colon. Be sure to obtain a formula with pancreatin in it. Swallow 1 to 2 tablets with each meal.

Herbal Combinations: My customers' favorite one is Super Colon Cleanse. You can ingest 1 teaspoon twice a day in a glass of water or juice. It contains psyllium husks with support herbs.

Constipation

Constipation often results from dehydration. You may solve the problem by simply drinking 6 to 8 glasses of pure water each day. Eliminate all drinks containing caffeine, because caffeine is a dehydrating agent and can make the problem worse. Use as many natural foods, preferably raw, as possible to increase fiber in your diet.

Acidophilus: These beneficial organisms provide B vitamins and create bulk in the intestine and colon. This often works like magic for a constipated child or adult. Take 1 capsule once or twice a day on an empty stomach or use the enteric coated tablets. Chewable tablets are available for children. You can give the liquid form to babies in water, juice, or formula.

Cascara Sagrada: This substance, which comes from the bark of a tree, relieves constipation in about 8 or 10 hours. Take 2 capsules before bedtime and you will have results by morning. I have known people with severe constipation who needed 4 to 6 capsules to get results.

Herbal Combinations: There are many combinations that work well for occasional use. Adults usually take 2 capsules before bedtime, but some individuals need 4 to 5 capsules. One combination, Super Colon Cleanse, is a powder with herbs and psyllium husks. A teaspoon in juice at night works great. Senna should not be taken on a regular basis because your body will gain a dependence on it and will have difficulty returning to normal functioning. In other words, it is wise to use these combinations for short periods only, while you get long-term results by changing your diet and fluid intake.

Magnesium: Magnesium draws water to the colon and makes stools softer. Like most people, you are probably deficient in magnesium anyway, so this nutrient will do more for you than relieve your constipation. Use 1 capsule or tablet two or three times a day.

Crohn's Disease and Ulcerative Colitis

These inflammatory bowel diseases are characterized by intestinal pain, diarrhea, and the malabsorption of nutrients. The incidence of such problems is increasing in cultures which consume the refined and high-fat diets such as are common in the United States.

By contrast, such problems are virtually nonexistent in countries where the people ingest a more primitive diet. Food allergies can also be a problem. Eat a natural food diet, completely eliminating refined sugar and grains. Drink 2 to 3 glasses of fresh vegetable juice every day. Drink plenty of purified or distilled water and try soluble fiber at bedtime. A deficiency in minerals can create serious problems, so you may want to take a mineral complex. The magnesium in the complex can help relax and soothe the colon.

Enzymes: You need these for the proper digestion of proteins. They also work as anti-inflammatory agents. Take 1 to 2 tablets or capsules with every meal.

Acidophilus: If you are taking antibiotics, this product is a must to normalize intestinal bacteria. Use 2 capsules twice a day on an empty stomach.

Stabilized Oxygen: This destroys bacteria and adds oxygen to the blood. Try 20 to 50 drops in juice or water twice a day.

Essential Fatty Acids: These are important for the health of the lining of the colon. Use 1 tablespoon of flaxseed oil daily or use a combination of other essential fatty acids such as primrose, black current oil, borage, or fish oils.

Aloe Vera Juice or Gel: This substance soothes the intestinal tract and promotes healing. Normally you drink 1/2 cup, morning and night.

Cat's Claw: This herb cleanses the intestinal tract and has anti-inflammatory properties. It is useful for most intestinal and bowel complaints. Use 2 capsules two or three times a day.

Depression

Depression is usually a biochemical problem and can often be solved with diet, exercise, and supplements. Some prescription drugs such as steroids, birth control pills, and tranquilizers can cause depression. Sugar, refined foods, alcohol, and cigarettes can also cause imbalances in the body that promote depression. A good multivitamin/mineral supplement is very important to start the healing process. A program of exercise is vital even though it may be hard to motivate yourself. Moreover, some excellent relaxation tapes are available. My favorites are the Hemi-Sync tapes named *Sleeping Through The Rain and Guide to Serenity.*

Magnesium and Potassium Aspartate: These two minerals together in aspartate form are energy producers and will help you feel good. When that happens, you can exercise, get things done, and feel more in control. Try 1 to 2 capsules three times a day.

B-Complex Vitamins: Depression is a major symptom of a B-vitamin deficiency. Look for a formula with at least 100 mg of B-6. Since B-12 is hard for our bodies to absorb, take B-12 in a sublingual tablet that dissolves under your tongue and goes right into your bloodstream.

Tyrosine: This is an amino acid that is a direct precursor to brain chemicals that determine mood and energy. It also helps produce dopamine which is usually deficient in people with depression. Take 1,000 to 2,000 mg twice daily.

GABA: This is another amino acid that has been called the "brain's natural calming agent." It inhibits over-stimulation of the brain. My favorite is one by Now Foods called GABA Mood Support with B-6.

Kava: This is nature's anti-anxiety herb. It brings a sense of calm and peace without impairing memory or concentration. Take 150 mg one to three times daily or use it in a combination with St. John's Wort.

St. John's Wort: This herb has been tested in many studies and has been found as effective as prescription antidepressants. It eases depression, anxiety, apathy, and insomnia. Use 300 mg of the extract three times a day. I know a few people who only need to take it once a day. St. John's Wort makes your skin sensitive to the sun so you may have to be careful not to stay out too long. Now Foods has a combination called St. John's Mood Plus which adds B vitamins, magnesium, kava, valerian, GABA, l-Taurine, and l-Tyrosine. It has been very effective for my customers who have tried it.

5HTP: This herb extraction forms the intermediate metabolite between the amino acid l-Tryptophan and serotonin. The lack of serotonin causes depression and insomnia. Try 50 to 100 mg daily. Taken in the evening, it usually helps you sleep.

Essential Fatty Acids: Many studies indicate that essential fatty acids stabilize mood and prevent mental illness, including depression. Diminished omega-3 fatty acid concentrations are associated with mood disorders such as bipolar disorder. Take 1 tablespoon of flaxseed oil daily or 4 to 6 capsules of omega-3 fish oil. It takes three to twelve weeks of supplementation to see the results.

Diabetes

There are two theories about the cause of diabetes. One is that adult-onset diabetes is linked to fat in the diet. Researchers have found that when diabetics adhere to a low-fat, high-fiber diet—that is, a vegetarian diet—they are often able to reduce or eliminate their use of insulin. As people around the world increasingly adopt meat-based diets, the occurrence of diabetes rises dramatically.

The second theory is that the incidence of diabetes has grown with the expanded consumption of sugar. Many years of research supports the fact that a "sweet tooth" will lead to a lifetime of poor health and premature death. A growing number of young children are being diagnosed as having diabetes. This is no doubt due to the fact that they get incredible amounts of refined sugar in infant formulas, sweet cereals, candy, pop, ice cream, cake, pie, pastry, and other "foods" high in sugar. Is it any wonder that children's pancreases are failing at a higher rate? This obsession with sugar leads to obesity in both adults and children and the extra weight is directly involved in diabetes. In addition to changing your diet and getting regular exercise, a good multivitamin/mineral supplement is a must. Because diabetes causes massive losses of nutrients such as the B vitamins and minerals like magnesium, zinc, and chromium, supplementation is a must. Dr. Julian Whitaker, in his book *Reversing Diabetes,* gives detailed information about diet, exercise, and supplements.

Type 2 diabetes (adult onset) can almost always be controlled through diet, weight loss, and exercise. If you are willing to address these areas, the condition may even be reversed. Monitor your diabetes carefully while you see what works. The following supplements can help rebuild and/or repair the pancreas:

Antioxidants: The higher the diet is in antioxidants, the lower the risk for diabetes. Vitamin E helps treat diabetes and prevents its complications. The recommended dose is 400 to 800 IU daily. Vitamin C neutralizes free radicals that can damage healthy cells. Take 1,000 to 3,000 mg daily. Beta-carotene is another antioxidant which is valuable in keeping cells healthy.

Gymnema Sylvestre: This substance stabilizes blood sugar and even helps to rebuild the pancreas so it can produce insulin. It normalizes cholesterol levels and lowers the need for insulin. It is supposed to work for type 1 and type 2 diabetics. The recommended daily dose is 400 mg.

Ginseng: Japanese research has shown that ginseng improves wound healing and promotes the formation of new blood vessels. American research found that American ginseng, given 40 minutes before a meal, produced a 20% reduction in blood sugar levels. However, ginseng taken with a meal did not bring these results. Take 500 to 3,000 mg of American, Korean, or Chinese ginseng 40 minutes before a meal, and test blood sugar levels to know whether to use more or less.

Alpha Lipoic Acid: One scientific study found that 600 mg twice a day lowers the need for insulin. It reduces the kidney and nerve damage that we often see in diabetes. It also decreased the fasting lactate and pyruvate, and increased insulin sensitivity and glucose effectiveness. Some alternative doctors suggest 50 to 100 mg daily, but researchers in a number of studies gave up to 800 mg a day to their patients. You may have to determine what works for you.

Glucose Metabolic Support: This formula from Now Foods helps reduce and moderate blood glucose levels. It contains Glucosol, an herbal extract which effectively lowers blood glucose levels. It also contains gymnema sylvestre, chromium, alpha lipoic acid, vanadium, magnesium, and selected B vitamins. This formula has been very effective, especially if a person makes dietary changes. Take 1 capsule with each meal. Recently a customer returned to my store the next day after buying this product to tell me that his blood sugar level had been 150 that morning instead of the usual 260, and that he had not needed to take insulin for three meals. Needless to say, he was delighted. Another customer told me that his blood sugar level had gradually declined every day until it had reached 150 after two weeks on the supplement.

Evening Primrose Oil: Diabetic neuropathy, a condition suffered by many diabetics, is a gradual degeneration of the nerves. The GLA present in Evening Primrose Oil has been shown to ease this affliction. Some studies showed that GLA combined with alpha lipoic acid worked even better. The full benefits may require up to six months of supplementation, so be patient. Take the product with food for better absorption.

Magnesium: Most diabetics have magnesium deficiencies. One study indicated that the lower the magnesium levels, the higher the risk of diabetic retinopathy. Extra magnesium can protect your eyes. Magnesium citrate or aspartate are the most absorbable. Take 200 mg two or three times a day.

Vanadyl Sulfate: Studies have shown that daily doses of 100 to 150 mg of vanadyl sulfate effectively reversed the diabetic condition, and when patients discontinued the vanadyl, the diabetic condition did not return.

Pycnogenol and Grape Seed Antioxidant: These are antioxidants which protect your blood vessels and capillaries from free radical damage. This makes them valuable for treating and preventing diabetic retinopathy. Take 1 milligram for every pound of body weight the first week, then half that dose thereafter.

Essiac: This herbal combination of sheep sorrel, burdock root, slippery elm bark, and Turkish rhubarb is normally used for cancer but it also helps diabetics. It seems to regenerate the ability of the pancreas to produce insulin. Drink 2 ounces twice a day on an empty stomach for two weeks to see if it works for you. If it does, you can continue it indefinitely.

Cinnamon: This herb helps stabilize blood sugar levels by improving glucose metabolism in fat cells by twenty fold. Take 1 teaspoon of cinnamon a day in juice or on oatmeal.

Diarrhea

The possible causes of diarrhea are many—food, medications, supplements, infections, stress, or a beginning health problem such as inflammatory bowel disease. If you get diarrhea, drink plenty of water, because diarrhea puts you at risk for dehydration. Bananas, rice, applesauce, and tea help solidify the stools, while foods like dairy products, fruit juices, spicy foods, fried foods, and junk foods make it worse. Some people are gluten-intolerant, and that condition can cause diarrhea. You may have to eliminate bread, pasta, or wheat products to see if one or more of them are causing the problem. A multivitamin/mineral supplement can replace nutrients that are being flushed out.

Grapefruit Seed Extract: Available in liquid or tablets, this is the first line of defense against any germ that causes diarrhea. The adult dose is 20 drops in juice or 2 tablets, but even a baby can receive 2 to 3 drops in juice. Never put it in your eyes, and do not use it full strength in your mouth.

Acidophilus: Taking 2 capsules of acidophilus on an empty stomach usually helps normalize your stools within 24 hours. You can give liquid or chewable tablets to babies and children. Another way to get acidophilus is to eat yogurt several times a day.

Zinc: In one study a deficiency in zinc resulted in diarrhea in 25% of the cases. Take 50 mg daily to see if it helps. The dosage for children is 10 mg and 5 mg for babies.

Diverticulosis

These little protrusions or sacs in the bowel sometimes become infected and inflamed. Long-term constipation often causes this condition. Eating more raw foods and getting enough water will help the problem. A multivitamin/mineral supplement can assist by supplying the nutrients needed for the repair and rebuilding of the walls of the colon.

Fiber: Use a source of fiber such as psyllium husk, oat bran, grapefruit fiber, or apple fiber. See which one works best for you.

Beta-carotene: It protects and heals the walls of the colon. Take 25,000 IU daily.

Acidophilus: Beneficial bacteria that help increase absorption of nutrients and improve elimination. Try 2 capsules one or two times a day on an empty stomach.

Essential Fatty Acids: You can take flaxseed oil, fish oil, primrose oil, or a combination. This is essential for healthy cells in the colon lining. Take 1 tablespoon of flaxseed or another oil, or the equivalent in softgels.

Cat's Claw: As an anti-inflammatory and cleanser, it reduces gastrointestinal symptoms. Try 1 capsule one to three times a day.

Green Grass Powder: You can use a teaspoon of barley or wheat grass powder in water or juice. Green grasses supply many nutrients needed to rebuild the health of the colon. It is even better to drink an ounce of freshly juiced barley and/or wheat grass.

Earaches

A rise in the incidence of ear infections has occurred as the use of refined foods has expanded. To solve the problem, increase the amount of raw food you eat and use unrefined breakfast products. Take a multivitamin daily. A doctor friend told me that he learned in medical school that the ear tubes which are put in children's ears cause constant ear infections. When children receive antibiotics for ear infections, some of the germs move to the ear tube and are not destroyed by the antibiotics. Then they can re-infest the ear canal and cause another infection. Because of this, you may want to think twice about getting tubes in your child's ears. Diet, supplementation, and treatment with herbs work well without causing more problems.

Nutribiotic Ear Drops: This product, which contains grapefruit seed extract and tea tree oil, works faster and better than anything I have ever tried. Placing no more than 2 to 3 drops in the ear usually calms the pain and allows the child to sleep. You can use it up to three times a day, but usually once or twice solves the problem.

Garlic Oil: A few drops of warm garlic oil in the ear is soothing and kills the microbes which produce earaches. I used this when my children were young and it usually worked. There are also garlic preparations with mullein and lobelia. Lobelia seems to help with the pain.

Colloidal Silver: A few drops of this in the ear often reduces the pain and accelerates healing.

Vitamin C: Vitamin C fights infection by enhancing the immune cells. Give 500 mg of chewable vitamin C to a child every hour for a few days until the earache is better. Then continue the child on vitamin C two or three times a day for a week or so to prevent a recurrence. Adults can have 1,000 mg every hour.

Ear Candles: When you burn an ear candle, it creates a suction which pulls the wax, fungus, candida, yeast, and other particles out of the ear and into the candle. The heat from the smoke is also soothing to the ear. Candles that have essential oils in them have extra healing power. My youngest daughter always asks me to candle her ears when she gets an ear infection, and that normally solves the problem. Instructions usually come with the candles.

Xylitol Gum: If your child has recurrent ear infections, you might try gum sweetened with xylitol. In a number of studies, xylitol reduced the germs which caused the earaches. Even chewing the gum seems to help.

Eye Problems

As you become older, your eyes may have problems adjusting to sudden darkness or glare. You may have difficulty reading small print or distinguishing faces at a distance. Cataracts and macular degeneration are becoming much more common. However, it is never too late to improve your eyesight with nutritional supplements.

Antioxidants: Studies have shown that people with higher intakes of antioxidants such as vitamins A, C, E, beta-carotene, and selenium have a lower incidence of macular degeneration. You can take a multivitamin/mineral supplement which contains all of them.

Bilberry: Bilberry contains compounds which help stabilize blood vessels and collagen in the retina, improves night vision and recovery from glare. Take 120 to 360 mg daily of the standardized extract.

Lutein: This is an antioxidant that is present in the macula (the center of the retina) of the eye. It absorbs the harmful ultraviolet radiation from sunlight and promotes macular health. However, since the amount of lutein decreases in the body as we age, it is important to take steps to increase its levels to help our eyes remain healthy. One way to do this is to take 15 to 20 mg of lutein daily. Lutein is found primarily in dark green, leafy vegetables such as spinach and collard greens. Eating an abundance of these vegetables will reduce your risk of experiencing macular degeneration. Some recent independent studies indicate that beta carotene interferes with the absorption of lutein so take vitamin A from fish oils if you are taking lutein in supplement form.

Glutathione: There is a strong relationship between glutathione and the aging of the lens of the eye. Low levels of glutathione is directly linked to cataracts, macular degeneration, and other eye problems. Glutathione levels also decline with age so supplementation is necessary when these problems appear. Usually 500 mg a day is adequate.

Taurine: Studies have shown that deficiencies in taurine lead to degeneration of the retina. Take 500 mg daily to protect your eyes.

Colloidal Silver: Spraying a solution of 15 to 20 parts per million of colloidal silver in the eyes reduces itching and dry eyes. You can also put one to two drops in each eye, but I prefer the spray.

Fatigue

The most common complaint I hear from people who come into Kathy's Herb Shop is their lack of energy. The solution is not the same for everyone. Sometimes the answer is as easy as taking a high potency multiple vitamin/mineral formula such as Eco Green or Special Two by Now Foods. Sometimes it takes a little experimentation to see what makes you feel more energetic.

Lack of energy is frequently the earliest symptom of such health problems as diabetes, anemia, cancer, hypothyroidism, allergies, malabsorption, hypoglycemia, poor circulation, and others. It is important to solve this problem so it will not develop into one of the more serious problems. Persistent fatigue is often the result of poor diet, especially when we eat refined foods and those high in fat. Other energy thieves are alcohol, caffeine, drugs, tobacco, stress, and incorrect eating habits. See the Life Choices section (pages 7-14) for more on diet and water.

A common cause of fatigue is dehydration. Carbonated and caffeinated drinks are one of the biggest causes of dehydration. It takes 8 ounces or more of water to process 8 ounces of this kind of drink, but rarely does anyone drink water after drinking the soft drinks. As a result, the body takes water from vital organs to process the chemicals in the drinks. This process leads to dehydration, lack of energy, stomach troubles, heart problems, and many other adverse conditions. Be sure to drink water when you first arise, 20 to 30 minutes before meals, and also between meals. It is not a good idea to drink water with meals as it dilutes the digestive fluids and interferes with digestion.

Another common reason for fatigue is an underactive thyroid. See the section on Thyroid (page 111) for instructions on how to test for this. The following products are used to increase energy:

Cayenne: This herb is a circulatory stimulant and works to make you feel better. Try 2 capsules with a meal.

HGH Preparations: These come in tablets or liquid. They help your body produce human growth hormone, which improves muscle strength, heart efficiency, and energy. My favorite is a homeopathic HGH from Liddell Labs.

Bee Pollen: Contains all known vitamins, 22 amino acids, 27 minerals, vitamins, and phytochemicals. Try taking 2 to 4 capsules daily for increased energy and endurance.

Spirulina and Chlorella: These are blue-green algae that contain a large amount of high-quality protein, carotenoids, B-12, vitamin E, easily absorbed minerals, essential fatty acids, chlorophyll, and much more. Take 6 tablets of spirulina (500 mg tablets) at lunch and another 6 with dinner. Chlorella often comes in 1,000 mg tablets so 3 with lunch and 3 with dinner is usually sufficient. Within a few days, you should feel more energetic both physically and mentally.

Magnesium and Potassium Aspartate: I recommend the aspartate form of these minerals for quick energy. Try 1 capsule up to three times a day.

Ginseng: This herb has been used for centuries to increase energy and well-being. Try 2 capsules once or twice a day.

B-12: Deficiencies of B-12 are common because this nutrient is hard to absorb as we get older. The vitamin plays a crucial role in energy metabolism, immune function, and the synthesis of DNA. Use the lozenges which dissolve under the tongue to facilitate the absorption of the B-12 into the blood. One or two lozenges a day (1,000 to 2,000 mcg) usually increases energy level in a few days.

Stabilized Oxygen: Oxygen is the best source of energy for all the cells in the body. Stabilized oxygen puts oxygen into the bloodstream quickly, where the cells can use it. There are several brands. I have used one called ION and it works for me. Take 20 drops in juice twice a day. I have also taken 5 drops under the tongue when driving on a long trip. It helped to revive me and keep me awake.

Olive Leaf Extract: If the fatigue is due to a virus such as Epstein Barr, olive leaf extract can usually help. Take 2 capsules of the extract twice a day and evaluate your progress after a month.

Maca: This herb works on your entire body to combat stress and fatigue while increasing energy and stamina. Take 2 capsules once or twice a day.

Fever

Fever is the body's way of attacking a disease by destroying the pathogens with heat. When a fever reaches 102 degrees or more, the body produces interferon in large quantities. Interferon is the strongest and most effective bacterial and viral medicine ever known. Do not take drugs to reduce the fever unless it goes above 104 degrees. The rare convulsion caused by a fever will not cause brain damage, and there is more risk in using aspirin or Tylenol than there is in having a convulsion. Take supplements to boost the immune system and thus enable the body to quickly deal with the cause of the fever. A garlic enema can aid in this process.

Vitamin C: Large amounts of vitamin C help to enhance the immune system. Take 250 mg of liquid vitamin C every hour for babies and small children, and 1,000 mg of vitamin C every hour for older children and adults.

Echinacea: This herb stimulates the immune system for faster recovery. Take a dropper full of the glycerine tincture three times a day for babies or children, and 2 capsules three times daily for adults.

Garlic: This has antibiotic properties and stimulates the immune system. Take 2 capsules three times a day

Fibroids and Endometriosis

Fibroids are growths (benign tumors) in the uterine wall. They have been linked to an underactive immune system and an overabundance of estrogen. The best way for women to prevent them is to improve their diet. Meat especially contains hormones which make this condition worse. Raw fruits and vegetables, and whole grains bind with the estrogen in the digestive tract to speed elimination. The raw juices of carrots, celery, and beets are very good and help cleanse the body. Use herbs that boost the immune system. See Cancer (page 60). Also, take a good antioxidant formula to reduce free radicals and to support the immune system. Drink plenty of pure water.

Vitamin E: It balances body hormones and scavenges for free radicals. Take 400 to 800 mg daily of D-Alpha tocopherol. If you see Dl-Alpha tocopherol on the label, it is synthetic and simply not effective.

Progesterone cream: Growths in the uterus are usually due to an oversupply of estrogen. Use progesterone cream, which normalizes body hormones and enables the body to dissolve fibroids, endometriosis, and other growths. I know a woman whose ovarian cysts disappeared while using the cream. Use as directed on the jar.

Essential Fatty Acids: These are needed to regulate and balance hormones. You can take omega-3 from fish oil, flaxseed oil, or primrose oil. Primrose oil is particularly good for this purpose. One tablespoon of the oil daily, 1 or 2 softgels of the 1,300 mg primrose oil, or 4 softgels of the fish oil is the usual dose.

Fibromyalgia

This disease brings chronic pain and usually affects the lower back, neck, and shoulders. The immune system is usually impaired so colds, flu, and other sickness are frequent. Drinking 8 glasses of pure water every day and consuming a diet of mostly raw foods will increase energy and reduce pain. Raw vegetable juices and 1 to 2 ounces of wheatgrass juice taken daily are very beneficial and will build up your immune system. People with this problem usually do not absorb nutrients well, so it would be beneficial to take a double dose of a good multivitamin/mineral supplement at every meal and extra amounts of vitamins E and C. Digestive enzymes are also needed to absorb the nutrients more efficiently.

Human Growth Hormone (HGH): People with fibro-myalgia are typically deficient in HGH. Liddell Labs has a homeopathic HGH that you spray under your tongue three times a day. Within a month you should notice a difference in how you feel.

MSM: This substance has anti-inflammatory and muscle-relaxing effects. Start with 1,000 mg daily and increase to 5,000 mg daily.

Magnesium Malate: This is a combination of malic acid from apples and magnesium. It is used for chronic pain. Most chronic pain sufferers are deficient in magnesium. Start with 1 tablet three times a day and increase if needed.

Bromelain: This is an anti-inflammatory substance from pineapple. Take as directed on the bottle.

CoQ10: This co-enzyme improves energy and circulation. Take 60 to 100 mg daily.

Fibro-X: This formula from Olympian Labs contains malic acid, shark cartilage, white willow bark, valerian, grape seed extract, magnesium glycinate, and manganese glycinate. It helps with pain and accelerates healing. Take 2 capsules with each meal.

Gallbladder

Gallstones are associated with a diet high in fat and refined carbohydrates, but low in fiber. This type of diet reduces the flow of bile acids, leading to the formation of gallstones. To resolve the problem, change to a natural diet of raw fruits and vegetables, and whole grains. Eliminate refined foods. Researchers have shown that casein (a protein) from dairy products increases the formation of gallstones in animals. On the other hand, vegetable proteins have a protective effect. Drinking 6 to 8 glasses of water each day can prevent gallstones from forming. You can often stop the pain of a gallbladder attack by drinking a tablespoon of apple cider vinegar in a glass of apple juice.

Silymarin: This active ingredient in milk thistle extract is a powerful liver detoxifier and improves the solubility of bile. Take 2 capsules a day with a meal.

Magnesium: This mineral makes calcium soluble and prevents gallstones. Customers taking magnesium for gallstone pain report less and less pain each day until it disappears. As long as they keep taking magnesium, the pain does not return. Take 1 to 2 tablets of magnesium citrate with meals two or three times a day.

Gallbladder Cleanse: If you decide to cleanse your gallbladder, choose a day when you have little to do because you will have diarrhea and pass stones all day. Do not eat or drink anything after 2:00 p.m. At 6:00 p.m. drink 6 ounces of water with 1 tablespoon of Epsom salts mixed in. At 8:00 p.m. drink another 6 ounces of water containing Epsom salts. At 10:00 p.m drink 1/4 cup of olive oil mixed with the juice of a grapefruit. However, make sure you go to the bathroom *before* you drink the olive oil. Then lie down immediately and try to go to sleep. The sooner you lie down, the more stones you will pass. When you awake in the morning, take another dose of the Epsom salts with water. You can go back to bed if you do not feel well. Two hours later, take another dose of Epsom salts with water. Two hours after that, you can eat some fruit. Eat lightly and by dinner you will probably feel fairly good. Gallstones are tan and green and they float. When you have a bowel movement, you may see up to 2,000 of them, of all sizes. You can repeat this cleanse every two weeks until you no longer see stones. The Epsom salts relax the muscles and ducts so that it does not hurt to pass the stones.

Gout

Gout is a type of arthritis caused by the buildup of uric acid in body fluids. The uric acid crystals migrate to a joint (usually the big toe) and cause intense pain. To treat this condition, avoid foods which produce uric acid—meat, sardines, mackerel, anchovies, and shellfish. Alcohol makes gout much worse, so you will have to eliminate it too. Drink plenty of distilled water to keep your urine diluted. This helps your body to excrete uric acid and prevent the crystals from forming. Eat whole grains and foods low in fat. It is helpful to drink 2 to 4 glasses of fresh vegetable juice each day.

Folic Acid: This B vitamin has been shown to inhibit the enzyme responsible for producing uric acid. Take the B-12 and folic acid lozenges under the tongue three or four times a day so it enters your blood stream rapidly.

Cherries: A half pound of fresh cherries, a handful of dried cherries, or an ounce of cherry concentrate can be eaten every day to lower uric acid levels and prevent the destruction of joints.

Quercetin: This flavonoid inhibits uric acid production, functioning like the drugs which doctors commonly prescribe for gout. Take 200 to 400 mg of quercetin with 1,000 to 2,000 mg of the enzyme bromelain two or three times a day between meals. Bromelain increases the absorption of quercetin so it is beneficial to take them together.

Hair

Bleaching, dyeing, perming, hot rollers and curling irons, and air dryers can damage your hair. Use natural hair products with nutritional support such as B vitamins, jojoba oil, chamomile, and other herbs. Hair that is dry or falling out needs nutrition. There are vitamin formulas specific for building up the health of your hair. They contain B vitamins and other nutrients (such as zinc) needed for healthy hair. Hair loss can also be caused by an underactive thyroid. See Thyroid (page 111).

Flaxseed Oil: Essential fatty acids are important in hair health. Using 1 tablespoon of flaxseed oil every day makes a noticeable difference within a month. The hair becomes softer and shinier and stops falling out in bunches.

MSM: Taking this biological sulfur can help stop hair loss and premature greying. Use 2000 to 4000 mg daily.

Headaches

Headaches can be caused by food allergies, eyestrain, muscle tension, poor posture, too little sleep, hormonal changes, caffeine, chemicals in food (aspartame and MSG), and stress. You may need to keep a record about what was happening before the headache to see if there is a pattern. Allergies to milk products, wheat, chocolate, food additives, and artificial sweeteners (aspartame) are the most common causes. If your neck or back is out of alignment, you may want to see if a chiropractor or a massage therapist can help. Dr. F. Batmanghelidj (see Resources, page 121, for his books) says that dehydration plays a major role in the precipitation of migraine headaches and that getting enough water will stop the mechanism that begins the headache. A lack of oxygen may also be a factor. Practice deep breathing morning and night to see if that helps.

Stabilized Oxygen: This puts oxygen into the bloodstream and usually lessens headache pain. Take 20 to 30 drops in water or juice.

Magnesium: Studies show that people with frequent headaches have low levels of magnesium in the brain and body tissues. A special kind of magnesium, magnesium malate, is for pain. Take this or magnesium citrate two or three times a day to see if it helps. You can take up to 1,000 mg a day in divided doses.

Feverfew: This herb is recommended for the prevention of migraine headaches. Take 150 mg daily for prevention.

Magnets: Magnets worn around the head with an elastic bandage really help some headache sufferers. You can experiment with where to put them.

Herbal Combinations: Combinations like Head Relief, Migra-X, and Headache contain feverfew and other nutrients that help headaches. These combinations sometimes are more effective than feverfew alone. Take as directed on the bottle.

Tiger Balm: Some of my customers obtain relief from headaches by rubbing a little of this ointment on their temples.

Heart

High blood pressure is usually the first sign that something is wrong with our circulatory system. It should be considered a serious warning for us to clean up our diet and get more exercise. Experts believe that free radicals are one of the primary causes of the buildup of plaque in the arteries. I suggest that people stop ingesting anything that creates free radicals, such as fried foods, overcooked or burned foods, chlorine, fluoride, other chemicals in culinary water, and nitrites in drugs and processed meats. The two countries that have the highest rate of heart disease, the United States and Finland, also have the highest consumption of pasturized dairy products, so it is vital that you eliminate or cut down on these foods. It is important to keep antioxidant levels high, to eat plenty of fiber-filled vegetables (preferable raw), and whole grains. Raw foods have substances in them that are natural, free radical fighters. Be sure to eat at least 3 raw foods a day (more is better) and include a carrot and a green salad. Celery is an important vegetable because it is a natural source of sodium and does not raise your blood pressure. Drink plenty of water. Sometimes just drinking 6 to 8 glasses of clean purified or distilled water a day, and eliminating all sodas and coffee, is enough to lower your high blood pressure. A study of 34,000 Seventh Day Adventists showed that people who drank a minimum of 5 glasses of water each day had half the risk of heart attack and stroke than those who only drank 2 glasses daily. If you take prescription heart drugs, I recommend that you read the book *Prescription Alternatives* by Earl Mindell and Virginia Hopkins. The authors review the dangerous side effects of various heart drugs and recommend safe alternatives to replace them.

If you find yourself alone and believe you may be experiencing a heart attack, there is a way to help yourself. Take a deep breath and then cough twice, as hard as you can. After a few seconds, take another deep breath and again cough hard twice. Continue this procedure until help arrives or your heart begins to beat normally. As soon as your heart stabilizes, take 1/2 teaspoon of cayenne pepper in warm water or 2 capsules with a glass of warm water. The technique just described is a method of self-CPR that was described in Dr. David Williams' newsletter called *Alternatives*.

Listed below are supplements which are useful in the treatment of high blood pressure, congestive heart disease, irregular heart beat, angina pain, and high cholesterol levels:

Coenzyme Q10: This is probably the most important heart nutrient for the circulatory system. It lowers blood pressure, oxygenates the heart muscle, and extends life for those with congestive heart disease. The natural production of CoQ10 by the body declines with age, so most people over 50 years old should benefit from it. The daily dose is 100 to 300 mg taken with a meal. CoQ10 is better absorbed in a small amount of fat, so take it with a meal that includes fat.

L-Carnitine: The function of this amino acid is to facilitate the transport of long-chain fatty acids. This prevents fatty buildup in the heart and circulatory system. The combination of L-Carnitine and CoQ10 for congestive heart disease is remarkably effective. The suggested dose is 1,000 mg one to three times a day. It is absorbed better on an empty stomach.

Cayenne: Cayenne is a circulatory stimulant and reduces cholesterol buildup. Dr. John Christopher, the famous natural healer, saved many heart attack victims by directing them to drink a cup of hot water mixed with 1 teaspoon cayenne. Take 2 capsules two or three times a day with meals or ingest cayenne powder by stirring1/4 to 1/2 teaspoon of the powder in a glass of water.

Hawthorne Berry: This herb strengthens and restores heart muscle. Clinical and laboratory research findings show that hawthorne may be beneficial in treating a number of heart conditions, including arrhythmia, angina, atherosclerosis, high blood pressure, and elevated cholesterol levels. Take 2 capsules two or three times a day, or take 1/4 to 1 teaspoon hawthorne berry syrup in combination with the cayenne.

Garlic: Garlic keeps cholesterol from accumulating on the walls of the blood vessels and maintains the elasticity of the arteries. Eat a clove a day or take 1 to 2 garlic capsules. There are deodorized products available if you do not want to smell like garlic.

ProFibe: This is a grapefruit pectin bound to guar gum and protein. It prevents the bad LDL cholesterol from turning rancid in your bloodstream and sticking to the artery walls. ProFibe can reduce cholesterol levels up to 25 to 30% in as little as a month. It works to reduce existing soft plaque and heals arteries. My customers claim that this product has produced a miracle for them. They report improved blood pressure, increased energy, and lower cholesterol in two or three months. You take 1 scoop of the powder in juice or water 1 to 3 times a day. There are 32 servings in each container.

Antioxidants: Since free radicals are thought to be the primary cause of plaque buildup in the arteries, taking antioxidants can neutralize free radicals before they cause damage. Vitamin C (1,000 to 5000 mg daily) is an antioxidant which reduces cholesterol levels and high blood pressure. It protects against blood clotting and promotes healing and repair. Vitamin E (400 to 1,000 IU daily) strengthens the immune system and heart muscle, improves circulation, and destroys free radicals. Beta-carotene and selenium are also important free radical fighters.

Magnesium and Potassium Aspartate with Taurine: This is a formula from Now Foods. Magnesium and potassium are minerals needed by the heart for energy and the proper regulation of the heartbeat. Magnesium relaxes the arteries and improves blood flow. Taurine is an amino acid which is essential for the efficient metabolism of sodium, potassium, calcium, and magnesium. It also inhibits the development of an irregular heartbeat.

Essential Fatty Acids: Omega-3 oils in fish oil or flaxseed oil boost the body's immune system, help normalize blood pressure, and reduce triglyceride levels. They also thin your blood and thus decrease the risk of blood clots. Take 1 to 2 tablespoons of flaxseed oil daily or the equivalent amount of flax or fish oil in softgels.

Conjugated Linoleic Acid (CLA): A free fatty acid that has decreased in our foods. By improving fat transport across cell membranes, CLA improves cardiac function at the most fundamental level. Try 2 softgels two or three times a day.

Ginseng: Several studies have shown that ginseng improves blood flow to the heart and reduces the stickiness of the blood platelets, which lowers the incidence of blood clots. Take 1 or 2 capsules daily. American and Korean ginseng are stronger than Siberian ginseng.

Stabilized Oxygen: In one study liquid oxygen was used to prevent heart damage after a heart attack. Fifty drops was the dosage. It helps prevent a heart attack when used regularly. Take 20 drops in water or juice twice a day.

Olive Leaf Extract: This is used for the normalization of heart beat irregularities and for the improvement of blood flow in cardiovascular and/or peripheral vascular disorders. Take 1 capsule of 18% oleuropein two or three times a day.

Homocysteine Regulators: This formula by Now Foods contains B-6, B-12, folic acid, and trimethylglycine. These nutrients aid the body's regulation of homocysteine, a potentially harmful byproduct of protein metabolism which damages the heart. One tablet a day is usually enough.

Lecithin: This is an emulsifying agent from soybeans which helps digest and remove cholesterol from the body, protecting it from fatty build up. Thus, it protects you against cardiovascular disease. You can obtain it in capsules, liquid, or granules. Take as directed.

Hemorrhoids

These swollen veins around the anus and in the rectum can be caused by constipation, obesity, lack of exercise, food allergies, diet, or pregnancy. This is another problem linked to the highly refined, low fiber diet eaten by most Americans. Eat more raw fruits and vegetables and drink 6 to 8 glasses of water every day. Swelling, bleeding, burning, inflammation, and irritation are among the unpleasant symptoms of hemorrhoids. Soaking in a hot bath usually relieves symptoms. Comfrey ointment is soothing and helps heal the tissues. Aloe gel applied to sore spots relieves pain and burning. Cream or lotion containing MSM is also soothing and reduces swelling.

Psyllium husks: Using 1 tablespoon of these husks in water or juice every day relieves hemorrhoids by making the stools softer and more bulky so you do not have to strain.

Flaxseed: Take 1/4 cup of ground flaxseed daily in juice or sprinkled on food. This promotes healing by making stools softer and providing essential fatty acids.

Vitamin E: Encourages healing and prevents scar tissue. Take 400 to 800 IU daily.

Vitamin C with Bioflavonoids: Builds the strength of the capillaries and veins and aids in healing. Take 1,000 mg three times a day.

People Paste: Use this as a poultice on sore spots. Cover with plastic wrap to prevent the paste from rubbing off, and leave it on all night. It lessens pain and speeds healing. See Natural and Herbal Recipes (page 119) for how to make it.

Hepatitis and Liver Problems

Hepatitis can remain dormant in the body for up to 30 years so by the time symptoms appear the liver may already be damaged beyond repair. Hepatitis C leads to more liver transplants than any other disease. Protect your liver by using a natural food diet and eliminating chemicals such as caffeine, alcohol, acetaminophen, and others which hasten the destruction of the liver. Drink plenty of water to help flush out toxins. The following remedies can help rebuild and protect the liver:

Alpha Lipoic Acid: A powerful antioxidant that is soluble in both water and fat so it can enter all parts of the cells. It boosts your levels of glutathione which the liver needs for detoxification. It also helps the liver receive energy from glucose so that it can restore itself. For serious liver problems the dose is large—200 mg three times a day.

Silymarin: Studies have shown that three to twelve months of treatment with this herb can result in a complete reversal of liver damage. It regenerates the liver by stimulating protein synthesis, neutralizing toxins, and raising glutathione levels by as much as 35%. Take 900 mg daily in divided doses.

Selenium: Decreases the replication of the hepatitis C virus and is a powerful antioxidant. Take 400 mg daily in divided doses.

Detox Support: A combination for cleansing the liver and blood. It contains silymarin, oregon grape root, dandelion root, red clover, beet root powder, MSM, bladderwrack, chlorella, selenium, copper, zinc, and manganese. Use as directed on the bottle.

MSM: A natural form of organic sulfur which is used in the body to assimilate methionine and cysteine and helps build new cells. New cells are what the liver needs. Start with 1,000 mg daily and increase to 3,000 to 5,000 mg.

Shark Cartilage: This substance has been used in programs to boost liver function. Take 1,500 mg daily.

Liver Extract or Concentrate: This comes in liquid or tablets. It stimulates liver cell regeneration. Take 1 tablet or a liquid dose a day for three months, then have a doctor check your liver function to see if it is working better.

Herpes

Genital herpes is the most prevalent sexually transmitted disease in the United States. It can range from a silent infection with no symptoms to a serious inflammation of the liver. Herpes can cause outbreaks of itching, burning, and fluid-filled blisters on the sexual organs of men and women. These sores are highly infectious and each outbreak can continue up to three weeks. Epsom salts baths can relieve the itching. You may accelerate healing by putting tea tree oil on the sores. Take a good multivitamin/mineral with zinc and B vitamins. Large amounts of vitamin C (5,000 to 10,000 mg daily) will help prevent the sores and inhibit the growth of the virus. Avoid peanuts and nutritional supplements containing arginine because they may cause outbreaks of the virus.

Herp-Eeze: This formula from Olympian Labs is very effective for treating herpes infections. Take as directed on the bottle.

l-Lysine: Inhibits the growth of the herpes virus. Take 1,000 mg morning and night.

Beta 1, 3 / 1, 6 D-Glucan: Stimulates the activity of the immune cells that digest invading bacteria and viruses. Take as directed on the label.

Olive Leaf Extract: Used in the prevention and treatment of human herpes viruses. Take 1 to 2 capsules three times a day for a herpes outbreak or 1 to 2 capsules a day for prevention.

Flaxseed Oil: The body needs this for any kind of skin outbreak. It promotes healing. Take 1 tablespoon of the oil or 4 to 6 capsules every day.

Moducare: This immune-enhancing product from Natural Balance contains sterols and sterolins from plants that increase the number and activity of the natural killer cells. Take 2 capsules three times a day until the sores are gone.

Hives

There are many possible causes of this allergic reaction—food, food additives, medication, infection, and even the antibiotics found in meat, dairy, and poultry. You may have to keep a record to track down what leads to the reaction. A good multivitamin/mineral can help by building your immune system and correcting any deficiencies that may contribute to the problem.

Acidophilus: Replaces the "good" bacteria and can reduce allergic reactions. Take 1 to 2 capsules on an empty stomach twice a day. Chewable tablets or liquid are available for children and babies.

Anti-Allergy formula: Now Food's Respir-All has nettle root, quercetin, and bromelain, all of which have anti-inflammatory properties. Take as directed on the label.

Zinc: Boosts the immune system and helps the skin heal. Take 50 mg daily.

MSM Lipsome Lotion: My customers tell me that this lotion by Now Foods is very effective for many types of skin problems. Take as needed.

Hormone Imbalance and PMS

A hormonal imbalance can lead to many problems for women of all ages. By consuming soy products, you can increase estrogen activity in the body. Eliminate refined carbohydrates and caffeine from your diet. Also, it is important to take a good multivitamin/mineral formula with at least 50 mg of B-6.

Wild Yam Progesterone Cream: Many women use this for the symptoms of PMS, menopause, and hormonal imbalance. It works to eliminate hot flashes, vaginal dryness, and balances your hormones so you can become pleasant to live with once again. Also, since progesterone is the single most important hormone necessary for the survival of the unborn child, drops in progesterone level or a blockage of progesterone receptor sites can result in a miscarriage. Many women who experience repeated miscarriages find that using the progesterone cream for the first 4 to 5 months of pregnancy prevents the premature loss of a baby. At about 3 to 5 months the placenta takes over the production of progesterone, and the woman can gradually discontinue the cream. Rub 1/4 teaspoon on alternating parts of your body. For instance, one night rub it on your stomach, the following night on your upper legs, and the third night on your upper arms.

Black Cohosh: Women in Europe use this as an alternative for estrogen. It is effective for hot flashes, insomnia, and depression in menopausal women. The recommended dose is 250 to 500 mg of the extract three times daily. It sometimes takes three or four weeks to start working.

Magnesium: Extra magnesium can help with problems of depression and lack of energy. Magnesium is necessary for the production of hormones. Take 600 to 1,000 mg daily.

Chaste Tree Berry: An effective therapy for PMS. In one study more than half the women found relief from bloating, breast fullness, headache, irritability, and mood swings. You can use this as part of a formula or take 2 capsules once or twice a day.

Dong Quai: A Japanese study showed that dong quai increased both estrogen and progesterone levels in women who had insufficient ovarian function. It can help with vaginal dryness and hot flashes. Take a combination that contains both black cohosh and dong quai.

Essential Fatty Acids: Necessary for hormone production. You can try flax oil, evening primrose oil, or fish oil.

Female Balance: This is a combination that contains B-6, folic acid, borage oil, wild yam, dong quai, and vitex agnus castus extract. Take as directed on the bottle.

Hypoglycemia

The symptoms of hypoglycemia include headaches, dizziness, trembling, depression, anxiety, irritability, a craving for sweets, and many others. The symptoms usually occur a few hours after eating sweets or high fat foods, but may occur much sooner. Stress can also be a factor. Hypoglycemia can also be an early sign of diabetes, so make dietary changes now. Eliminating sweets, high fat foods, caffeine, and refined foods are necessary to get well. Use lots of raw foods and a vitamin/mineral supplement daily.

Chromium: This trace mineral works with insulin to carry glucose into the cells. Without chromium, glucose levels are elevated. Take 200 mcg daily to balance blood sugar.

Essiac Tea: Several customers tell me that as long as they use essiac tea every day, they do not experience an attack of hypoglycemia. Therefore, the tea seems to balance blood sugar levels. Take 2 ounces once or twice a day. See Natural and Herbal Recipes section (page 117) on how to make it or buy prepared liquids or capsules.

Protein Powder: Using more protein sometimes helps to maintain energy levels. My favorite protein powder is Rice Protein from Nutribiotic because the processing never heats the product above 90 degrees F. As a result the protein is not denatured by heat.

Impotence

The inability to maintain an erection may result from the use of over-the-counter or prescription drugs, diabetes, alcohol, cigarettes, circulatory problems, hormonal imbalances, or psychological is-sues. If your arteries are clogged to the extent that there is a blockage in blood flow, see the section on Heart (page 84) for some possible solutions. Most cases of impotence have a physical cause, so you may have to change your diet, initiate an exercise program, and take antioxidants and a good multivitamin/mineral supplement.

Ginseng: People have used this herb for hundreds of years to improve their stamina and longevity, in both sexual matters and general health. The Panax, American, and Korean ginsengs contain more of the active ingredient than Siberian ginseng. Take 2 capsules once or twice a day or drink the herb made into a tea.

Biogra: This formula from Olympian Labs contains a mix-ture of vitamins, minerals, and herbs that are known to increase performance and endurance. Take as directed on the bottle.

Mascutone: This product by Dr. Christopher's Original For-mulas contains herbs to strengthen penile health and function. They recommend 2 capsules three times a day.

Yohimbe: An herb from the bark of a West African tree. It opens the veins of the penis, allowing more rapid and rigid erections. It also enhances libido and the intensity of the sexual experience in men. It can cause anxiety or nervousness in some people and is not recommended for men with high blood pressure or those on antidepressants.

L-Arginine: Supplementing with this amino acid increases blood flow to the penis, resulting in harder erections with more staying power and frequency. Take 3 to 6 grams of l-Arginine 45 minutes before sexual relations.

Essential Fatty Acids: These precursors of hormones are nec-essary for the formation of sperm and the health of the prostate. Take 1 tablespoon daily or 4 to 6 softgels.

Ginkgo Biloba: Medical research indicates that this herb is able to increase blood flow throughout the body, including the penis, and it can be more effective for impotency problems than medically prescribed drugs. Take 160 mg of the extract with meals three times a day. Results are usually seen in a few weeks but improve within three months.

Androstene: This supplement is responsible for the develop-ment of the male sex drive and libido. It promotes muscle growth while maintaining adequate levels of testosterone. If you have been diagnosed as having too little testosterone, this is the product that may help. Take as directed on the bottle.

Incontinence

Loss of bladder control may occur at any age, but it is more common in people over fifty. It often results from weakened pelvic muscles, infection, pregnancy, spinal cord injury, or neurological dysfunction. In men it can also be due to prostate inflammation. See Prostate (page 107). Alcohol and caffeine may be culprits in this problem. Use more raw foods and take a good antioxidant formula. Vitamins A, C, E, and zinc can also help.

Calcium and Magnesium: These minerals work to control bladder spasms in some kinds of incontinence. Magnesium relaxes muscles and helps the body to utilize calcium. Try 200 mg of magnesium citrate three times a day and 1,000 mg of calcium daily.

Homeopathic Combinations: Such as Hyland's EnurAid incontinence tablets. Take as directed.

Super Kegal Exerciser: This exerciser fits between your thighs and you depress and relax 10 to 20 times. This strengthens weak pelvic muscles. Weak pelvic muscles are the cause of stress incontinence, a condition where urine leaks when you cough, sneeze, laugh, or lift a heavy object.

Indigestion and Flatulence

Many people have problems with digestion and flatulence, especially as they get older. When we are young, we usually eat junk foods which create a strain on our bodies. As a result, our digestion does not function properly when we become older. Taking a digestive enzyme with meals usually helps people who have difficulty digesting their food. Now Foods has a product called Super Enzymes, designed to help people assimilate protein, carbohydrates, and more. Usually you take 1 to 2 tablets with meals, but I have one customer who has to take the pills twenty minutes before eating to get good results.

Soft drinks may also create problems with digestion. These cold drinks lower your stomach temperature, which lessens the effectiveness of the enzymes, puts stress on the digestive system, and hinders proper digestion. Undigested food often causes gas. If you are constipated, it probably shows that you are dehydrated. When you are dehydrated, digestion is not complete. Drink 6 to 8 glasses of purified or distilled water every day and you will see some positive changes in your body, including increased energy. Another cause of flatulence is parasites. Undigested food is a great source of nourishment for parasites (which most of us have), and you may have to take a parasite cleanse to destroy the parasites. Grapefruit seed extract works wells for many different kinds of parasites.

Apple Cider Vinegar: A tablespoon of apple cider vinegar after each meal increases stomach acid to assist digestion. If the vinegar causes you distress, you probably already have enough acid and should not use the vinegar.

Acidophilus: Taking acidophilus for a month or two puts the "good" bacteria back into the digestive system and can make a big difference. Take 1 to 2 capsules a day on an empty stomach.

Activated Charcoal: This can absorb many times its weight in gas. Take 2 capsules or tablets with meals. Be aware that your stool will be black, but it is just the charcoal.

Stabilized Oxygen: The pH of our stomach becomes more alkaline as you grow older, causing digestive problems. This allows putrefactive bacteria to develop, and these bacteria create gas. Oxygen kills anaerobic bacteria (those which thrive in environments without oxygen). Take 20 to 50 drops of the liquid in juice every three or four hours for a few days to destroy the bacteria.

Clay Liquid: Taken every day for two or three weeks, this product absorbs toxins and balances the intestinal tract with minerals. See Natural and Herbal Recipes (page 119) for how to make it.

Cayenne: This herb has the ability to clear the blood of matter and gasses that cause digestive problems. To avoid burning in your stomach, you might take it as a tincture (a dropperful in a little water with each meal), or take 1/4 teaspoon of the powder in water with a meal.

Tumeric: This herb aids digestion, and reduces bloating and gas. Sprinkle a little on your meal or take one capsule with a meal.

Infertility

Many factors can cause infertility. Fluoride and chlorine affect fertility in most animal species, including humans. To avoid this problem, consider purchasing a water purifier. Other types of chemicals also affect fertility. Mercury exposure (from silver teeth fillings) has been found to cause hormone disturbances which lead to reduced fertility. The use of alcohol and tobacco reduces sperm count and can prevent the implantation of an egg. To avoid or treat infertility, improve your diet. Eliminate junk foods and eat more fruits, vegetables, whole grains, and nuts. A good multivitamin/mineral formula would be beneficial. Make sure it contains selenium and zinc. A selenium deficiency has been linked to infertility in both men and women. Zinc is essential for reproduction. If the infertility results from hormonal deficiencies, see Hormone Imbalance and PMS (page 91).

Vitamin E: Breeders give this vitamin to prize animals that cannot conceive. Also, it works well for humans. Vitamin E is needed for hormone production and increases sperm count in men. Both the husband and wife should take 400 to 800 IU daily.

Vitamin C: Keeps the sperm from clumping and makes them swim faster. Try 1,000 mg three times a day.

Maca: This herb has been used for 500 years for increasing fertility. Take 2 capsules twice a day for a few months.

Lycopene: This is a natural plant carotenoid commonly found in tomatoes. In a study of 50 men with low sperm counts who received lycopene supplements twice a day for three months, 36% of the men later fathered children.

Influenza

The symptoms of flu begin the same as a cold—coughing, hot and cold sweats, fatigue, headache, and body aches. This is followed by a fever and sometimes nausea and vomiting. When the flu hits, stay in bed and rest. Use juices, soups, and drink plenty of liquids because these take less energy to digest.

Grapefruit Seed Extract: This is my favorite for the flu. I have gotten rid of the vomiting and nausea in a few hours by using this as early as possible. My favorite is the Maximum Strength GSE which also contains vitamin C, mushrooms to boost the immune system, echinacea, ginger, goldenseal, yarrow, and zinc. Liquid is also available for children and for those who have a hard time swallowing tablets.

Zinc C Lozenges: If you are low on zinc, the flu or a cold can seem to last forever. The immune system needs zinc to fight viruses. Use the lozenges every two hours at the first sign of a cold or flu. My favorite one is Zinc-C by Now Foods because it does not have a metal aftertaste. Elder-Zinc, another product of Now Foods, adds elderberry, which has antiviral properties and reduces flu symptoms.

Colloidal Silver: Good for viral infections. Adults take 1 teaspoon two or three times a day. Children take 1/4 to 1/2 teaspoon according to weight, twice a day.

Vitamin C: Whenever my children were sick, I would give them as much chewable vitamin C as they would take. Because of that, they were not sick very long. Vitamin C boosts the immune system by increasing the number of white blood cells that attack the germs. Adults can take up to 10,000 mg daily in divided doses. Children can take the 500 mg chewables 6 to 8 times a day.

Insect Bites and Stings

Most insect bites are fairly harmless, but the itching and swelling may require some doctoring. Tick bites can spread disease, so if your child has a tick, remove it with tweezers as soon as possible and treat the puncture with Miracle Oil, tea tree oil, or People Paste. If you take B vitamins, they will make you smell bad to mosquitos, so it would help if you gave everyone B vitamins every day for a week or two before you go on a camp out. You will attract mosquitos if you eat refined sugar products because you will smell sweet. Perfume, hair spray, cosmetics, and bright colors also attract insects. To repel insects, buy a natural bug repellent or make your own with essential oils. See the appendix on Natural and Herbal Recipes (page 119).

Miracle Oil: I have used this mixture of essential oils on wasp stings, mosquito bites, tick bites, and itching lumps of unknown origin. It reduces the swelling and pain. See Natural and Herbal Recipes (page 118).

DMSO: People use this liquid for bites by recluse spiders and other kinds of insects. It reduces swelling and speeds the healing.

Tea Tree Oil: It disinfects and soothes insect bites.

People Paste: I have used this on mosquito bites, spider bites, and wasp and bee stings with excellent results. It decreases the swelling and heals the wound faster. Just spread the paste over the bite, cover it with plastic and tape, and leave on up to twelve hours. Reapply the ointment if needed, but usually that is not necessary. See Natural and Herbal Recipes (page 119) for how to make it.

Quercetin and Bromelain: A bioflavonoid and enzyme combination which diminishes allergic reactions. Take 200 to 400 mg every four hours until the swelling and inflammation disappear.

Insomnia

It is estimated that up to forty million Americans suffer habitually from insomnia. Habitual sleeplessness has many possible causes—physical illnesses, depression, stress, pain, medications (antidepressants, antiseizure medication, beta-blockers, decongestants, thyroid replacement drugs, and appetite suppressants), caffeine, and nutritional deficiencies. A lack of calcium and magnesium can keep you from sleeping. Over-the-counter sleep medications can cause depression, dry mouth, drug dependence, and a worsening of the insomnia. These drugs prevent the deep sleep cycles which the body needs to feel rested. Do not forget exercise. A good exercise program, done faithfully, can help the body establish proper sleep patterns. Also, relaxation and meditation tapes are available which can produce long-term results. Hami-Sync produces some excellent tapes called *Sleeping Through the Rain and Guide to Serenity.* To soothe and relax your body and mind, take a warm bath with ten drops of lavender oil in it before bedtime. A hot cup of tea like chamomile or a relaxing tea blend is very effective for some people.

Calcium and Magnesium: Take up to 1,000 mg of calcium citrate and 1,000 mg of magnesium citrate in divided doses with your meals. Since magnesium is a nerve nutrient and muscle relaxant, take 200 mg at bedtime. These two minerals will help you sleep and prevent nighttime leg cramps and twitches.

Melatonin: This is a natural hormone that promotes sound sleep. Some authorities believe we should take melatonin occasionally or our bodies will stop their own production of this hormone. Certain drugs like beta-blockers or aspirin can lower the body's melatonin levels and supplementation may be necessary. Take 1 to 5 milligrams one hour before bedtime. Use the lowest dose that helps.

Valerian Root: Clinical tests have shown that this herb promotes sleep without causing morning grogginess. It quiets and relaxes your entire body. Take 2 capsules one hour before bedtime or use it in a formula with other relaxing herbs. My favorite is Nighttime Herbs Extract from Now Foods which contains kava, chamomile, passion flower, catnip, hops, and valerian.

5HTP: This is an extraction from an African herb that is the intermediate metabolite between the amino acid l-Tryptophan and serotonin. Serotonin is needed for sleep and relaxation and this substance enables the body to make it. Use 50 to 100 mg before bedtime.

Menopause

Premenopausal and menopausal symptoms are usually a result of an imbalance between the body's levels of estrogen and progesterone; the amount of estrogen rises while that of progesterone decreases. This can cause your menstrual cycle to be irregular and your periods heavier and longer. You may experience hot flashes, mood swings, headaches, heart palpitations, anxiety, insomnia, vaginal dryness, weight gain, and fatigue. See Hormone Imbalance and PMS (page 91).

Black Cohosh: Black cohosh is used to alleviate premenopausal and postmenopausal symptoms including hot flashes, depression, emotional fluctuations, and insomnia. Research shows that 40 mg of the root extract of black cohosh is very effective in alleviating the symptoms of menopause.

Essential Fatty Acids: They are essential for the production of body hormones. Evening primrose oil, black current oil, and flaxseed oil are good sources of essential fatty acids.

Vitamin E: Reduces hot flashes and other symptoms of menopause. Take 400 to 800 IU daily in divided doses.

B Vitamins: These anti-stress vitamins help prevent mood swings and fatigue. Take a B complex such as B-50 once or twice a day.

Soy Isoflavones: They contain a form of estrogen and work to eliminate hot flashes and other symptoms. Take 2 capsules a day.

Metal Toxicity

Our bodies are exposed to many toxins in our air, water, and food. We have mercury in our tooth fillings, lead in our bones from leaded gasoline, and many other chemicals and metals from breathing polluted air and drinking treated water. Signs of toxicity include headaches, fatigue, sluggish thinking, weight gain, poor digestion, and muscle pain. Chronic fatigue syndrome is often a sign of toxicity in the body. Eliminate cigarettes, alcohol, and refined food. Organic food puts much less stress on the body, allowing it to eliminate metals and toxins. To help the body heal itself, drink 6 to 8 glasses of pure water daily.

The body does not eliminate metals such as aluminum and mercury easily. Since metals will bind with sulfur in the body and are then eliminated, it is important to increase sulfur in the body. Cilantro is one of the highest sulfur bearing plants and using 1 bunch of cilantro either in a salad or juice every day will help the body get rid of metals. Soaking in high sulfur mineral springs, using sweat baths once or twice a week and using MSM will also help. Using this program, I eliminated 90% of a high blood concentration of aluminum in seven weeks.

Spirulina: Japanese researchers have shown that spirulina protects the body against mercury and drug-induced kidney failure. This makes it valuable for people suffering from the effects of silver dental fillings.

Alpha Lipoic Acid: This is used in Europe as a oral chelating agent in the treatment of heavy metal toxicity. Take 200 mg once or twice a day.

Liquid Clay: Clay passes through the intestinal tract undigested, and as it does so it collects heavy metals, pesticides, and chemicals, and removes them from the body. Take this product for two or three weeks. You can buy it in liquid form, or see Natural and Herbal Recipes (page 118) to make it.

Vitamin C: Protects the body from metal poisoning. Take 1,000 mg twice a day

Methylcobalamin: A type of B-12 that is deficient in people who suffer from metal toxicity. If you take 1 mg daily in a lozenge dissolved under the tongue, it should increase your energy and sense of well-being.

MSM: Since this is biological sulfur, it will combine with metals in the blood and then be flushed out of the body. I increased the MSM to 6,000 mgs a day when I was detoxing from aluminum.

ANTI-TOX METALS: This homeopathic formula from Liddell Labs is an antidote for exposure to the toxic metals aluminum, mercury, dental fillings and water pipes. Use as directed on the label.

Multiple Sclerosis

The cause of this progressive, degenerative disorder of the nervous system is not known but there are educated theories. Some experts think there is a virus involved. Others implicate pesticides, chemicals, or heavy metal poisoning. A few researchers link MS with mercury from tooth fillings because MS sufferers have seven times more mercury in their system than healthy people. To treat or prevent this disorder, I suggest that you eat organic foods, and eliminate chemicals and all animal foods. Use mostly raw vegetables and fruits and drink 8 glasses of pure water daily.

Selenium and Vitamin E: MS patients are deficient in these antioxidants. Adding them to their diet corrects these deficiencies and decreases the symptoms.

Grapeseed Extract or Pycnogenol: One of my customers with MS says this is what helps her the most. She takes 120 mg daily.

Methylcobalamin: A type of B-12 that is needed in the brain. In one study of patients with chronic, progressive multiple sclerosis, 60 mg daily produced an improvement in visual and auditory function. For best results take it with Alpha Lipoic Acid. Lozenges to put under your tongue are available in doses of 1 mg and 5 mg. You might try taking the 1 mg lozenges three times a day or 1 to 2 of the 5 mg lozenges.

Nausea

The main causes of nausea in most people include motion sickness, pregnancy, and flu. In the pregnant woman it is dehydration which usually produces this condition. If you have this problem, drink more water. If a glass of water makes you sick, take small sips all day long. Squeezing a little fresh lemon juice in the water can help you drink more. Take 1 tablespoon of apple cider vinegar with each meal to facilitate the absorption of the B vitamins in your food. This normally solves the nausea problem.

Ginger: Try chewing on a piece of fresh ginger. However, if that is too strong, take crystallized ginger instead, but in this case you will get some sugar also. Another possibility is to take ginger capsules every three hours. Some people find that ginger tea works for them.

Peppermint oil: This essential oil, which you apply to your neck, wrist, or a drop on the tongue, can help with nausea incidental to pregnancy, an illness, or car sickness.

Magnesium: Settles the nerves and relaxes muscles. Take 200 mg of magnesium citrate for car sickness one hour before a trip.

Liquid B Complex Vitamins: You may relieve nausea due to pregnancy or motion sickness by placing some vitamin B liquid, such as Total B, under your tongue. This is more effective if you use it as soon as the nausea starts. Take as directed.

Vitamin B-6: A lack of B-6 can cause nausea, but sometimes taking it makes you feel sick and results in vomiting. A product from Now Foods, P-5-P, is an enteric coated B-6 which passes through your stomach and is absorbed by the body in the intestines. Because it bypasses the stomach, it usually prevents nausea. Use 1 tablet once or twice a day.

Homeopathics: People use nux vomica and veratrum album either separately or together for nausea due to pregnancy or other causes. Put 3 pellets of each under the tongue as needed.

Obesity

A recent study of one million patients, reported by the New England Journal of Medicine, found that overweight people ran a higher rate of premature death, even if they did not smoke and considered themselves healthy. The study also discovered a clear association between excess weight and a higher risk of dying from heart disease or cancer.

If you are determined to lose weight, do not follow one of the current diet plans in vogue. They will nearly always disappoint you in the long run. Instead, make a complete and permanent change in your living habits. First, change the way you eat. Eliminate refined sugar and starches, throw the junk food out of your house, and do not bring it home anymore. See the chapter on Natural Diet (page 7). Second, drink lots of pure water—at least 8 glasses a day. This helps to hydrate the body and makes it easier to lose weight. Third, exercise at least five times a week. Spend a minimum of twenty minutes riding a bike, jumping on a trampoline, walking briskly, or whatever other vigorous exercise you enjoy doing.

L-Carnitine: This amino acid is found in most weight loss combinations because it transports the long-chain fatty acids to the mitochondria, increasing energy production. Take two 500 mg capsules once or twice a day. When my clothes started getting too tight, I went on a juice fast for a couple days and added 2 capsules of L-carnitine every day to prevent weight gain. It worked for me.

Conjugated Linoleic Acid (CLA): This free fatty acid helps you take off pounds by increasing your body's metabolic rate. As a result, your appetite decreases and more fat cells are consumed in the production of energy. In a recent study in Norway, people taking 3 to 4 grams of CLA a day achieved significant body fat reductions.

Calcium Pyruvate: This can improve both fat and weight loss by increasing metabolism and fat utilization. The usual dose is 2 to 4 tablets, one to three times daily on an empty stomach.

Spirulina: A blue-green algae that is a concentrated source of minerals, vitamins, and protein. It is used by dieters as an appetite suppressant. Take 6 tablets before lunch and 6 before dinner.

Maca: This herb reduces your body's rate of converting carbohydrates into fats, acts as a natural appetite suppressant, and reduces the production of fatty acids in metabolism. Take 1 to 2 tablets before a meal.

Chromium: This mineral balances your blood sugar so that you do not crave sweets. When you are deficient in this mineral, your cells cannot properly absorb the glucose needed for energy. You can get it in a multiple vitamin/mineral formula or take 50 to 100 mcg daily.

Chitosan: This fiber from shellfish binds to fats during digestion and reduces their absorption. Take 1 to 2 capsules when you eat a meal with a lot of fat. Do not take it with every meal because you need some fat in order for your body to function properly.

Osteoporosis

Osteoporosis is a disease of calcium deficiency, yet Americans ingest more calcium than people in other countries where the incidence of osteoporosis is low. The greatest cause of osteoporosis is eating too much protein. Americans consume about five times as much protein as people in other countries. Excessive protein creates an acid environment in the digestive tract and the body has to compensate by using minerals to make it more alkaline. If the minerals are not available, your body takes them from your bones. I know several older people who take a great deal of calcium in supplements, but whose bone density tests do not improve. However, if they changed to a mostly raw food diet and seriously reduced the quantity of animal protein they consume, they would enjoy better health and more efficiently absorb the calcium they get.

Also, people should take calcium citrate or calcium aspartate, because the body absorbs them quite easily. Since magnesium is necessary for the utilization of calcium, they need to get plenty of it. Boron, taken with calcium and magnesium, slows down calcium loss in the urine.

In women, the problem of osteoporosis is compounded by a lack of hormones. They can compensate for this by applying a wild yam progesterone cream everyday. This can correct a progesterone deficiency so that calcium is absorbed more efficiently. European studies demonstrate that women regain bone loss with the daily use of wild yam progesterone cream.

Magnesium: Calcium cannot be absorbed without magnesium, and 87% of Americans are deficient in magnesium. Take magnesium citrate or aspartate for best absorption. It is probably sufficient to take 200 mg three times a day. Leg cramps often respond to increased magnesium intake.

Ipriflavone: This substance from soy inhibits bone resorption. Also, it increases bone density by enhancing bone formation. Take 300 mg twice a day.

Essential Fatty Acids: Recent research shows that animals deficient in essential fatty acids develop severe osteoporosis and increase deposits of calcium in their kidneys and arteries. Essential fatty acids increase calcium absorption, reduce urinary excretion of calcium, and increase the amount of calcium deposited in the bone. One to two tablespoons of flax oil or a combination of flaxseed oil, evening primrose oil, and borage oil can make a difference in how you utilize your calcium.

Parasites

Parasites do not thrive in your digestive system when you eat a raw food diet. In fact, they tend to be flushed out. You should regularly eat foods like carrots, pumpkin seeds, pomegranates, raw onions, and raw garlic. My grandmother wormed her dog by shoving a clove of garlic wrapped in a piece of bread down the dog's throat. It worked very well, because the worms came out in the dog's stool the next day. Doing a parasite cleanse works better and faster if you combine it with a colon cleanse.

Grapefruit Seed Extract: I have customers who have used this to get rid of pin worms in their children. Also, I know of two babies who were diagnosed with Giardia and this is what worked for them. Take 2 to 3 drops of the liquid in juice for a baby, 5 to 10 drops in juice for a child, and 20 drops for an adult.

Black walnut tincture: The tincture should be made with the green hulls of the black walnut. Take 30 drops twice a day for an adult to kill worms. Use less for children.

Cloves: This herb kills the parasite eggs. Take 2 capsules three times a day for a week. You can grind your own whole cloves by powdering them in the blender; then you know they are fresh.

Olive Leaf Extract: Has been shown to be effective in killing a variety of parasites, including microscopic protozoa and macroscopic helminth worms. Take 1 capsule three times a day of the 15% oleuropein olive leaf extract, or 2 capsules three times a day of the 6% oleuropein.

Liquid Clay: Clay passes through the body and removes parasites and other matter from the intestines. Take for 2 or 3 weeks. See Natural and Herbal Recipes (page 118), for how to make it.

Parasite Formulas: Formulas like PARA-X by Nature's Way and Wormwood Combination by Kroeger Herb are used 2 to 3 times a day for a month to kill parasites.

Parkinson's Disease and Nerve Neuropathy

Parkinson's disease results from the destruction of the brain cells which use the amino acid L-dopa to produce dopamine. The medical treatment for this condition is to supply the patient with L-dopa and another substance called Carbidopa. However, the problem with this approach is that it leads to the release of glutamate, which causes the further destruction of brain cells, so eventually the treatment stops working. At the Whitaker Wellness Center (www.drwhitaker.com) they use an entirely different approach. They supply patients with intravenous glutathione to slow the process of nerve cell degeneration. This therapy meets with surprising success, even when Parkinson's disease has been established for years. If you cannot find a doctor who is willing to administer this amino acid therapy, you could take oral doses of glutathione. Try 1 to 2 capsules or tablets twice a day. Another promising treatment is the use of methylcobalamin, a form of B-12. It seems to slow the progression of nerve damage, and even produces nerve regeneration in some cases. In some studies, 60 mg of this substance was given by injection daily. In the supplement form, methylcobalamin is only available in 1 mg and 5 mg tablets, so that dosage could become expensive. Since the body has difficulty absorbing this substance, it comes in lozenges that dissolve under the tongue to get into the blood. Other studies suggest using 5 to 20 mg of this supplement daily.

Grape Seed Extract or Pycnogenol: Contains a powerful antioxidant known to cross the blood-brain barrier to neutralize free radicals in vital brain and nerve tissue. Take 100 to 200 mg daily in divided doses.

Pneumonia

Pneumonia has over 30 different causes, including bacteria, viruses, fungi, and chemical irritants. People with weakened immune systems are at the greatest risk. Fluid accumulates in the lungs in infected, pus-filled air sacs, limiting the body's ability to absorb oxygen.

Antioxidants: Take 5,000 mg of vitamin C daily in divided doses. After symptoms have disappeared, reduce the dosage to 3,000 mg a day and then to 1,000 mg for maintenance. Take 400 to 800 IU of vitamin E to prevent scar tissue and promote healing.

Magnesium: Acts as an antihistamine to keep air passages open. Take 200 mg of magnesium citrate twice a day.

Stabilized Oxygen: Puts oxygen in the blood stream when the lungs are having trouble breathing. Take 50 drops twice a day in juice or water.

Herbal Lung Formula: One formula is Nature's Way CL-7 which contains the lung-healing herbs mullein, chickweed, marshmallow, slippery elm, white pine, elecampane, and hyssop. Take 2 capsules twice a day.

Miracle Oil: Use 10 drops in a vaporizer to help clear breathing passages or you can take 2 to 3 drops internally in a small amount of water or juice. See Natural and Herbal Recipes (page 119) for how to make it.

Zinc: After reviewing ten studies, investigators report that zinc supplementation reduces the risk of pneumonia by 41%. If you have had pneumonia, it would be a good idea to supplement with 50 mg of zinc daily to prevent a recurrence.

Prostate

Approximately 75% of men over age 50 have an enlarged prostate. As the prostate gland enlarges, it constricts the urethra, causing frequent and incomplete urination. Sometimes urination becomes painful. A good multivitamin/mineral supplement can help.

Saw Palmetto: In nine different studies, saw palmetto extract was effective in the treatment of prostrate enlargement. Some natural healers suggest that men in their 40's should begin using saw palmetto to prevent prostate enlargement, even before symptoms appear. Usually 160 mg of the extract is enough but you can take up to 320 mg if needed.

Pygeum: This herb is also effective for enlarged prostate. It reduces swelling and works well with saw palmetto. The recommended daily amount is 100 to 200 mg of the standardized extract.

Stinging Nettle: Studies show that the standardized extract of stinging nettle increases urinary flow rates and reduces residual urine levels. Take 120 mg daily.

Essential Fatty Acids: Use a combination of EPA and GLA such as omega-3-6-9 by Now Foods. This is more effective for prostrate problems than just flax or fish oil, which only has the omega-3s. Take 2 softgels two or three times daily.

Lycopene: This carotenoid from tomatoes is an antioxidant which reduces the risk of cancer. You need about 3 mg daily.

Zinc Picolinate and B-6: Zinc is an important nutrient, and B-6 increases the absorption of zinc. Take 30 to 60 mg of zinc daily with a multivitamin that contains B-6.

Prostate Formulas: There are several formulas available from manufacturers which combine most of the above supplements. Most of my customers prefer the convenience of the formulas.

Sciatica

In his book *How to Deal with Back Pain and Rheumatoid Arthritis,* Dr. F. Batmanghelidj notes that back pain is often caused by dehydration of the spinal discs and the area surrounding them. This dehydration forces the surrounding muscles to work harder, and spasms result. Batmanghelidj states that 6 to 8 glasses of water daily are crucial to maintain healthy levels of water in our bodies. He adds that lower back pain often progresses into sciatic pain because of the displacement of a disc. He provides corrective exercises which actually put the disc back into place and strengthen your back. If you have back pain, this book may be a lifesaver.

Cayenne Ointment: This preparation is very effective for all types of muscle pain. Rub it on your sore back and buttocks, cover it with plastic wrap, and then put your underwear back on to hold it into place. Leave it on all night. It will feel hot for several hours, but in the morning you should feel better. You can repeat this procedure every night as long as you have pain. One good product for this purpose is Professor Cayenne's Deep Heating Rub.

DMSO Cream or Gel: This preparation helps remove pain from the muscles of your back. Just apply it to the areas which ache.

Magnets: Some people receive relief from pain by bandaging a flat magnet around the area which hurts. Some experts believe that the energy from the magnets alters the chemical interactions in the nerve fibers which are causing the pain. Others feel that the magnet increases blood flow to the area. The magnet should be the strength of 500 to 1,000 gauss.

Shingles

The elderly have an increased risk of acquiring this herpes zoster infection. Experts associate it with a diminished immune system. See Cancer (page 60) for immune system builders.

Antioxidants: Take 5,000 mg of vitamin C, 400 mg of B complex, 400 IU of vitamin E, and 50,000 IU of beta-carotene daily. Antioxidants boost the immune response and make the course of the infection shorter.

Nervine Tonics: Nervine herbal formulas can help soothe and nourish the nerves and accelerate healing. Take as directed on the bottle.

Cayenne Ointment: This will reduce the pain of the sores.

Nelson-Bach Flower Rescue Remedy™/Traditional Flower Remedies' Calming Essence™: Using 3 or 4 drops under the tongue every few hours will help relieve the emotional trauma of dealing with shingles.

Herp-Eeze: This formula from Olympian Labs was developed specifically for herpes infections. It reduces pain and accelerates healing.

Sinusitis

This is the most common chronic disease in the United States. Sinusitis may be triggered by a cold, allergies, air pollution, smoke, or stress. A natural diet and supplementation are important in fighting this infection. Use the following infection-fighting herbs:

Garlic: Contains antimicrobial compounds to fight infections. You can eat a whole clove of raw garlic, chopped and put on food, or use 2 capsules or tablets two or three times a day.

Echinacea: Stimulates the immune system to fight viruses or bacteria. Take 1 to 2 capsules morning and night.

Olive Leaf Extract: Several of my customers say this is what made them better. They took 2 capsules twice a day.

Skin Problems

Skin rashes can be caused by chemicals in the air or water, food allergies, and nutritional deficiencies. It has been found that 75% of children's rash cases result from allergic reactions to peanuts, milk, or eggs. Most skin problems, including eczema and dry skin, respond to essential fatty acids. Take omega-3 from fish oil, primrose oil, flaxseed oil, or a combination. Within a month you will probably see considerable improvement. Antioxidants, specifically vitamins C, E, and selenium help prevent changes in the skin that can lead to premature wrinkles and skin cancer.

MSM Cream or Lotion: My customers tell me this works best for healing all sorts of rashes and reducing the itching and pain. You can also take MSM internally for good results. Use 2,000 to 4,000 mg daily.

Spirulina or Blue-green Algae: A super food containing a wide variety of the vitamins and minerals which are the foundation for healthy skin. Take 3 to 6 tablets or capsules with meals two or three times a day.

Grape Seed Extract: A powerful antioxidant with known skin-preserving properties. Try 100 mg daily all at once or in divided doses.

Lactobacillus: Tests reveal that acidophilus taken regularly decreases eczema outbreaks by 50% in young children. Take it once or twice a day on an empty stomach. Use liquid or chewables for children.

Sore Throat

Sore throats are usually caused by a virus or bacteria and are often the first symptom of a cold or other sickness. See Colds (page 65).

Zinc Lozenges: Sucking on one of these every hour soothes and promotes healing, and usually gets rid of the sore throat within a day or two.

Sore Throat Juice: This is made from cayenne, vinegar, honey, grapefruit seed extract, and water. To heal your throat quickly, sip this preparation through a straw every five to ten minutes. I have never had to continue this treatment more than a day. See the Natural and Herbal Recipes (page 120) to see how to make it.

Miracle Oil: Get quick relief by swallowing 2 to 3 drops. You can also take 2 to 3 drops in a little juice or water if you feel it burns too much to use straight.

Colloidal Silver: A powerful natural antibiotic. Take as directed.

Thyroid

Hypothyroidism (underactive thyroid) is a growing problem. It is estimated that nearly 10% of us have undiagnosed thyroid problems. Symptoms include fatigue, constipation, muscle cramping, hair loss, weight gain, and joint pain. You can do your own home test to see if your thyroid is working normally. When you wake up in the morning, put a thermometer in your armpit and leave it there for ten minutes. Stay in bed while you wait. Record the results. A normal reading is 97.2 to 98.2° Fahrenheit. A reading outside that range generally indicates a thyroid imbalance.

Liquid Kelp or Dulse: This contains iodine, which nourishes the thyroid gland. Take 4 drops a day for a month and then 2 drops a day for maintenance.

Kelp Tablets or Powder: Some people prefer to take the tablets or the powdered form instead of the liquid. One customer told me that after half of her thyroid gland was removed, she found she could not take the prescription drug for hormone replacement. However, after taking 1 teaspoon of kelp powder every day in juice or water, her energy levels soon returned to normal.

Thyroid Glandular: If the kelp or dulse does not reduce the symptoms, take 1 tablet of thyroid glandular every day for three months. This helps rebuild the tissues of a genetically weak thyroid so it can utilize the iodine from kelp and function normally.

Tinnitus

The symptoms of tinnitus are the constant or intermittent sensation of noise such as ringing, buzzing, or hissing in the ear.

It can usually be heard only by the affected person. The causes include medications, chemicals, ear wax, perforated tympanic membrane, or exposure to loud noise. It occurs in 85% of people who have a hearing loss. A good vitamin and mineral supplement with extra C, E, magnesium, and potassium can really help.

Ginkgo Biloba: Studies in Germany confirm that the standardized extract of this herb is effective in the treatment of tinnitus. The amount used was 480 mg daily. This is the equivalent of eight 60 mg capsules daily or you could take 4 double-strength capsules. After a few months you might cut back on the dosage and see if you maintain the results.

Vitamin A: Studies show that a shortage of vitamin A leads to disorders of the inner ear. Try 25,000 to 50,000 IU daily and reduce to 25,000 IU after a few months. Beta-carotene can be used instead of vitamin A from fish liver oil because there is less toxicity associated with that form of vitamin A.

Tooth Decay and Gum Problems

Streptococcus mutans is the bacteria that lives in the plaque in our mouths and uses the sugar we ingest to produce the acid that causes cavities. Eating lots of refined sugar helps them to multiply rapidly and destroy our teeth faster. Tooth brushing and even flossing does not do the whole job. You can do a more complete job of brushing by using a water irrigator that flushes particles from between your teeth and the deep pockets in your gums. I also put 10 drops of grapefruit seed extract into the irrigator's water tank to kill the bacteria in my mouth. Health authorities link gum disease to other problems, such as heart disease, stroke, and susceptibility to infections. Bacteria in the mouth can enter the bloodstream through diseased and bleeding gums, travel throughout the body, and cause low-grade infection and chronic inflammation. Because of this, it is very important to take care of your teeth and gums. Be sure to brush your tongue, because that is where a lot of the harmful bacteria collect.

CoQ10: Specialists link deficiencies of this nutrient to periodontal disease. Coenzyme Q10 reduces inflammation and other symptoms of gum disease. Take 60 mg daily. One customer told me that her dental hygienist reported that the pockets around her teeth were large and needed cleaning often. After taking CoQ10 for six months, she returned to the hygienist, who now indicated that the pockets had shrunk to half of what they were, and her gums were much healthier.

Antioxidants: Vitamins C, A, selenium, and zinc are important for gum health. These nutrients prevent gum disease, inhibit plaque growth, and hasten healing. Gums that bleed easily when you brush your teeth are usually deficient in vitamin C. You can try an antioxidant formula that contains all these nutrients.

Herbal Tooth Pastes and Powders: There are some good antibacterial toothpastes that work well. Herbal Tooth Powder from Dr. Christopher is a combination of comfrey root, oak bark, horsetail grass, peppermint, lobelia, and cloves. It looks green when you brush, but it makes tooth enamel stronger and helps prevent gum disease. Other good toothpastes contain neem oil, olive leaf extract, echinacea, grapefruit seed extract, and other herbs.

Miracle Oil: A drop or two of Miracle Oil on your toothbrush (with or without toothpaste) will disinfect your mouth and kill tooth decay germs. It makes your mouth feel clean and helps heal gum disease. To make Miracle Oil, see Natural and Herbal Recipes (page 118).

Xylitol: A sweetener used in chewing gum. Since cavity-causing bacteria cannot properly digest xylitol, no acids form. The sweetener impairs the bacteria, which are flushed down the throat and destroyed by stomach enzymes. If you or your children chew gum, make sure it is sweetened with xylitol because it will help prevent tooth decay. Nature's Life has a chewable grape-flavored vitamin C that is sweetened with xylitol.

Ulcers

There are many factors which promote the formation of ulcers—bacteria, hyperacidity, stress, drugs, and certain kinds of foods. Using aspirin and other over-the-counter drugs, alcohol, or cigarettes increases your risk of developing ulcers. You can dilute excess acid and lessen the problems it causes by drinking 8 glasses of purified water every day. Fried foods, refined foods, and soft drinks make things worse by interfering with digestion. Drink raw vegetable juices like carrot, cabbage, and celery. Eat more foods raw and try to deal with the stress in your life. If you take vitamin C, use the buffered forms or Ester C so that it will not be acidic on your stomach. Take a multivitamin/mineral supplement to supply B vitamins, vitamin A, zinc, and other nutrients that are important for healing and handling stress.

Acidophilus: This repopulates your gastrointestinal tract with the good bacteria that help digestion and the assimilation of nutrients. Take 2 capsules three times a day on an empty stomach or take enteric-coated tablets with meals.

DGL Licorice: Deglycyrrhizinated licorice increases the mucous coating of the esophageal lining, helping it to resist the effects of stomach acid. Take 2 chewable tablets of DGL licorice before meals or between meals. I have a customer who takes 2 tablets before he goes to bed at night to prevent waking up with an acid stomach. With DGL licorice he can sleep all night.

Vitamin E: Helps heal and relieves pain. Take 400 to 800 mg daily with meals.

Apple Pectin: Soothes and coats the stomach lining to protect against stomach acid. Take 2 capsules with each meal.

L-Glutamine: An amino acid that is important for healing muscle tissue. Take 500 mg daily on an empty stomach. Amino acids are absorbed better on an empty stomach.

Liquid Clay: This is very healing if it is taken daily for two to three weeks. The clay passes through the body undigested and absorbs toxins as it passes. To make it, see Natural and Herbal Recipes (page 118).

GI Support: This preparation from Now Foods contains nutrients known to support the gastrointestinal tract, including DGL Licorice, apple pectin, L-Glutamine, MSM, cat's claw, enzymes, and aloe vera concentrate. Take as directed on the bottle.

Aloe Gel: Some of my customers drink 1/4 cup of aloe gel when their stomach hurts. Aloe is very effective in soothing and healing the stomach lining.

Varicose Veins

You have a better chance of getting varicose veins if you sit or stand for a long time. I suggest that you take regular breaks in order to exercise your leg muscles. Lie on a slant board with your feet up for thirty minutes a day to assist the flow of blood back to your heart. Use garlic, onions, and red pepper in your food. Compounds in these foods break down the fibrin which causes the lumpy skin around the varicose veins.

Horse Chestnut: This herb contains aescin, which enhances the structure and tone of veins and helps relieve the symptoms of fatigue, heaviness, pain, and swelling in the legs. It also works for nighttime leg cramps. Take 150 mg twice daily.

Bromelain: An enzyme from pineapple that breaks down fibrin. Use raw pineapple or 500 mg tablets three times a day.

Butcher's Broom: A time-honored treatment for varicose veins. Participants in studies experienced significant reduction of leg pain, swelling, and itching after two months on butcher's broom. They took 2 capsules three times a day of vitamin C.

Flax Seed Oil: Anytime body tissues are in trouble, you need to take essential fatty acids. The oil makes your veins more pliable and healthy. Use 1/4 cup of ground seeds daily or 1 tablespoon of the oil.

Warts

Warts sometimes disappear by themselves within six months to five years, but we usually want to speed the process. I have tried all kinds of remedies, such as treating a wart with the sticky white matter from the stem of the dandelion flower or visualizing the wart disappearing. If you have many warts, it is an indication that you need to boost your immune system. Try some of the immune builders under Cancer (page 60).

Grapefruit Seed Extract: Place a drop of the undiluted liquid on the wart and cover it with a band-aid. I even got rid of a plantar wart that was hard and painful. I soaked it, scratched away some of the hard skin, and applied the grapefruit seed extract and a Band-Aid. It was not until two weeks later that I realized it was gone.

Appendix 1
Natural and Herbal Recipes

Ear Wax Softener
1/2 teaspoon baking soda
2 ounces water
   Mix together. Drop 3 to 4 drops in your ear three times a day. In four to five days the wax should be soft enough to flush out with a syringe.

Essiac Herbal Formula
6 1/2 cups burdock root (cut)
1 pound sheep sorrel (cut or powdered)
4 ounces slippery elm bark (powdered)
1 ounce turkey rhubarb root (powdered)
   Mix herbs thoroughly together. To make the tea, use 2 gallons distilled or purified water in a stainless steel pot and 1 cup of the essiac herbal formula. Bring to a boil and boil ten minutes with the lid on. Allow to sit for 12 hours (stir after about six hours) and bring to a boil again. Then turn off the heat, strain, put in canning jars, and seal. Store in refrigerator. You can make half the recipe with 1/2 cup of the herbal mixture and 1 gallon of water.

Lemon/Olive Oil Drink
   This recipe is taken from the book *How to Reverse Immune Dysfunction* by Mark Konlee. Into a blender, cut up 1 whole lemon, rind, and pulp. First, be sure to wash the lemon well and scrape off markings from artificial coloring. Add 1 and 1/2 cup of fruit juice (such as orange juice), and 1 tablespoon of extra virgin olive oil (cold pressed). Blend at high speed for one minute. Pour through a strainer to remove pulp. Use a spatula to press the pulp. Discard the pulp and divide the resulting drink into 2 or 3 portions. Drink a portion with each meal or all at once. Taking it before bedtime can help you sleep. This drink helps detoxify your liver, balances pH in the saliva, restores nutrient absorption, deactivates HIV virus, reduces swollen lymph nodes, and stimulates white blood cells.

Liquid Clay

2 teaspoons Bentonite clay (powdered)
8 ounces purified water

Mix together and let sit for 12 to 24 hours. Do not touch or mix clay in metal. Clay has a negative charge and metal is positively charged, and you do not want to interfere with the clay's ability to draw out metals, toxins, chemicals, etc. from the intestinal tract. Take 1 glass a day for two or three weeks. You can mix a quart at a time by using 3 tablespoons of clay to a quart of water. The clay cure has been used for parasites, diarrhea, constipation, allergy, heartburn, indigestion, ulcers, acne, virus infection, spastic colitis, and food poisoning. It absorbs toxins and provides minerals to the body and is one of the most effective natural intestinal detoxifying agents available.

Miracle Oil

1 ounce cinnamon oil
1 ounce clove oil
1 ounce eucalyptus oil
1 ounce lemon oil
1 ounce rosemary oil

Mix all of these essential oils together and pour back into the one-ounce bottles. I use Now oils because they are pure and economical. I carry one bottle in my purse for occasional bug bites and sore throats that sometimes appear when I am away from home.

Natural Insect Repellant

5 drops citronella oil
5 drops lavender oil
5 drops geranium oil

Mix each oil together in 1 cup of distilled water. Put into a spray bottle and spray on arms, neck, face (close eyes) and any bare parts of the body. You can also put these drops into 4 ounces of oil such as almond oil or apricot seed oil, and rub on exposed parts.

People Paste

Mix equal parts of goldenseal, comfrey root, lobelia, and slippery elm powders. Store in a closed jar. When needed, take 1/2 to 1 teaspoon of the powder and add a little water (purified or distilled is best) to make a paste. Put paste on the sore or wound and cover with a little square of plastic to keep it moist. You can cover that with a bandage, elastic bandage, or just tape it on. Leave on for twelve or more hours. Use for bug bites, infection, and boils.

Raw Tahini Treats

1 cup honey or use 1/2 cup honey and 1/2 cup barley malt syrup
1 cup raw tahini or raw almond butter
2 cups raw nuts and seeds ground up in the blender (almonds, flax seed, sesame seeds, sunflower seeds, pumpkin seeds, etc.). For example: 1 cup sunflower seeds, 1/2 cup flax seeds and 1/2 cup sesame seeds. I always make it with at least 1/2 cup flax seeds.
1 teaspoon vanilla
1 cup unsweetened coconut
1 cup raisins or chopped dates
1 cup grain sweetened or date sweetened carob chips (optional)
1 cup chopped nuts (optional)

Warm the honey so that it is a liquid. Remove from the heat. Add tahini or almond butter and mix. Add the rest of the ingredients. Stir and knead until it is mixed together. Press into a plate or pan and cut in squares or form into a roll and store in a plastic bag in the refrigerator. Cut or break off pieces as desired. You can vary the recipe by adding wheat germ, lecithin, protein powder, popped amaranth, or nutritional yeast in place of some of the ground nuts and seeds. I even made it once using powdered spirulina. I liked it, but everyone else thought it looked unusual because it was green. Do not be afraid to experiment. I make it a little different every time. This is what I eat when I crave sweets.

Shara's Mouth Wash

1 quart water
25 drops peppermint oil
20 drops tea tree oil
10 drops grapefruit seed extract
5 drops Miracle Oil
3 drops myrrh oil (optional)

    Mix together, keep in a closed jar, and use for soreness or irritation of gums, fresh breath, or to disinfect mouth and teeth.

Sore Throat Juice

1 tablespoon honey
1 tablespoon apple cider vinegar
1/4 to 1/2 teaspoon cayenne powder or 2 droppers full of tincture
20 drops grapefruit seed extract (liquid)
8 to 10 ounces water

    Dissolve the honey in a few ounces of hot water, add cayenne powder, vinegar, and 20 drops of grapefruit seed extract. Add from 8 to 10 ounces of water. Stir. Take a sip every five to ten minutes until sore throat is gone. It is easier to sip it through a straw because then it does not burn your whole mouth, just your throat. This usually gets rid of a sore throat in two to eight hours. It is very soothing for coughs and works for laryngitis.

APPENDIX 2
RESOURCES

Web Sites

www.shirleys-wellness-cafe.com This is a big web site that discusses the health issues of men, women, children, and animals. It has a large number of links to other sites for further information.

www.fedbuzz.com/vaccine/vac.html A searchable database for adverse vaccine effects.

www.notmilk.com If you need some incentives to stop using dairy products, this is the most complete assortment of articles on milk products relating to health.

www.living-foods.com The largest site for raw food articles, information, and lots of recipes.

www.hoptechno.com/book11.html Tells how to start a personal fitness program and how to measure your heart rate in relation to exercise.

www.wellnessgoods.com Has some great information about water, meditation, and healing.

www.herbalhealer.com/breakingnews.shtml Special up-to-the-minute reports on health issues such as microwave ovens that you will not see on television.

www.dorway.com An intensive information site for aspartame. It covers how to tell if your health problem is linked to aspartame and what to do about it, plus lots more.

www.meatstinks.com Tells how to switch to a vegan diet, how to help change your school's cafeteria diet, and how to feed your dog or cat a vegetarian diet.

Books and Tapes

Balch, Phyllis A. and James F., MD, Prescription For Nutritional Healing, Avery, 2000. A practical A to Z reference to drug free remedies using vitamins, minerals, herbs, and food supplements.

Batmanghelidj, F., MD, *ABC Of Asthma, Allergies And Lupus*, Global Health Solutions, 2000. This book explains the direct relationship between water deficiency in the body and asthma, allergies, and lupus.

Batmanghelidj, F, MD, *How to Deal With Back Pain and Rheumatoid Joint Pain*, Global Health Solutions, 1991. A new approach involving the important role of water in holding the spinal column together. It also contains an exercise approach for displaced discs and sciatic pain.

Batmanghelidj, F., MD, *Your Body's Many Cries For Water*, Global Health Solutions, 1999. A complete water cure program for arthritis, back pain, heartburn, migraine headaches, heart disease, asthma, diabetes, and more.

Byers, Dorie, *Natural Body Basics: Making Your Own Cosmetics,* Gooseberry Hill Publications, 1996. Contains natural recipes for almost every hair and skin product imaginable.

Carroll, Lee and Tober, Jan, *The Indigo Children*, Hay House, 1999. Tells you how to recognize if you have an indigo child and how to raise him/her.

Coulter, Harris L., *Vaccination, Social Violence and Criminality: The Medical Assault On The American Brain*, 1990.

DeVries, Herbert, PhD, *Fitness After 50*, Charles Scribner's Sons, 1987.

Emoto, Masaru, *Messages From Water,* HADO Kyoikusha, 2000. Includes hundreds of incredible pictures of crystals from the experiments with water.

Hay, Louise L., *You Can Heal Your Life,* Hay House, 1999. How to restructure your life to find self-esteem and self-love. Has affirmations for healing, personal growth, and a great deal more.

Jensen, Dr. Bernard, *Dr. Jensen's Guide To Better Bowel Care*, Avery, 1999. A complete program for tissue cleansing through bowel management.

Kelder, Peter, *Ancient Secret Of The Fountain Of Youth*, Doubleday, 1998. This book contains the complete description of the five simple exercises that help to restore youthful health and vitality.

Konlee, Mark, *How To Reverse Immune Dysfunction*. 2000. An entire program for AIDS and HIV sufferers. Also covers chronic fatigue syndrome, candidiasis, and other immune related conditions.

Mindell, Earl L., PhD and Hopkins, Virginia, MA, *Prescription Alternatives: Hundreds of Safe, Natural, Prescription-Free Remedies To Restore and Maintain Your Health*, Keats Publishing, 1999. You can look up the prescription drug you are taking to find out the side effects and safe alternatives for replacement.

Myss, Caroline, PhD, *Why People Don't Heal And How They Can*, Harmony Books, 1997. A practical approach to healing life issues and overcoming the mental and emotional blocks to becoming well.

Price, Joseph, Dr., *Coronaries/Cholesterol/Chlorine*, Jove Publications, 1981.

Shinn, Florence Scovel, *The Game Of Life And How To Play It*, DeVorss and Company, 1925. Shows how positive attitudes and affirmations can make you a "winner" in life.

Ticciati, Laura and Ticciati, Robin, PhD, *Genetically Engineered Foods: Are They Safe? You Decide*, Keats Publishing, 1998.

Truman, Karol K., *Feelings Buried Alive Never Die...*, Olympus Distributing, 1991. Tells you why you feel the way you do and how to transform negative feelings so they do not hinder your growth.

Walters, Clare, *Aromatheraphy: An Illustrated Guide*, Element Books, 1998.

Weil, Andrew, MD, *Breathing, The Master Key To Self Healing*, Sounds True, 1999. A two tape set to help you learn the art of healthy breathing.

Whitaker, Julian, MD, *Is Heart Surgery Necessary?* Regnery Publishing, 1995. Tells how to eliminate heart medications and heal yourself naturally.

Wolverton, B.C., PhD, *How To Grow Fresh Air*, Penguin Books, 1996. Tells how houseplants can purify the environment by filtering toxins and adding moisture and oxygen to the air.

Index

A

acid 19, 23, 40, 42, 43, 49, 51, 55, 58, 59, 61, 62, 63, 64, 70, 72,
    81, 82, 83, 85, 87, 92, 93, 95, 99, 103, 104, 106, 112, 113, 114
acidophilus 52, 53, 63, 65, 67, 68, 69, 74, 90, 95, 110, 114
acne 39, 40, 118
activated charcoal 95
ADD 47-50
ADHD 47-48
affirmations 37, 122, 123
aging 7, 34, 40, 55, 76
AIDS 41, 42
air pollution 15-16, 109
alfalfa 45
alkaline 41, 95, 104
allergies 7, 13, 28, 42, 43, 48, 64, 69, 77, 83, 88, 109, 110, 122
aloe 59, 65, 69, 88, 114
alpha lipoic acid 40, 41, 55, 72, 89, 100, 101
aluminum 55, 57, 100, 101
androstene 93
anemia 43, 77
animal 11, 19, 20, 24, 25, 26, 31, 61, 81, 96, 101, 104, 105
antibiotic 19, 20, 52, 53, 54, 63, 65, 69, 75, 79, 90, 111
antioxidants 40, 41, 50, 60, 71, 73, 76, 86, 93, 101, 107, 109,
    110, 113
apnea 28
apple cider vinegar 39, 43, 52, 81, 95, 102, 120
arnica 59
arthritis 14, 44, 45, 82, 108, 122
aspartame 17, 18, 83, 121
asthma 7, 13, 18, 20, 28, 30, 42, 45, 46, 122
Attention Deficit Disorder 47-50

Attention Deficit Hyperactive Disorder 47- 48
autism 27, 28, 49, 51, 52

B

Bach Flower Remedies 50
Bach Flowers 44, 109
bad breath 52
bee pollen 41, 78
beta carotene 76
bilberry 76
black cohosh 91, 92, 99
black walnut 63, 105
bladder infection 52, 53
boils 54, 119
brain 9, 11, 18, 22, 27, 42, 47, 49, 50, 52, 54, 55, 56, 61, 70, 79,
    84, 101, 106
breast 11, 19, 56, 57, 58, 61, 62, 91
bromelain 42, 44, 46, 64, 81, 83, 90, 98, 115
bronchitis 58
burns 59
butcher's broom 115

C

caffeine 18, 19, 53, 57, 64, 68, 77, 83, 88, 91, 92, 94, 98
calcium 10, 11, 19, 49, 59, 61, 81, 87, 94, 98, 103, 104, 105
calcium pyruvate 103
Calming Essence™ 50, 109
cancer 8, 10, 11, 12, 13, 14, 19, 20, 21, 22, 23, 28, 40, 41, 56,
    57, 60-63, 65, 73, 77, 80, 103, 108, 109, 110, 115
candida 63, 75
carpal tunnel 64
cascara sagrada 67, 68
cat's claw 69, 74, 114
cavities 11, 12, 112
cayenne 46, 58, 78, 85, 86, 95, 108, 109, 111, 120

chemicals 7, 10-17, 20, 21, 23, 25, 56, 60, 67, 70, 77, 83, 84, 88,
    96, 100, 101, 110, 112, 118
chitosan 104
chlorine 11, 12, 14, 84, 96
chlorophyll 43, 78
chromium 40, 71, 72, 92, 103
cinnamon 73, 118
CLA 87, 103
clay 67, 95, 100, 106, 114, 118
cloves 105, 113
cold sores 64-65
colds 65-66, 80
colloidal silver 43, 51, 53, 75, 77, 97, 111
colon 8, 17, 22, 23, 52, 61, 66, 67, 68, 69, 74, 105
colostrum 66
comfrey 46, 59, 88, 113, 119
constipation 33, 43, 67, 68, 74, 88, 111, 118
cooking 8, 14, 21, 22
coQ10 61, 81, 85, 112
crib death 28
Crohn's Disease 68

D

dehydration 13, 18, 46, 65, 67, 73, 77, 83, 102, 108
depression 11, 17, 18, 34, 47, 49, 69-70, 91-92, 98-99
DGL licorice 114
diabetes 7, 28, 71, 72, 77, 92
diarrhea 16, 18, 68, 73-74, 82, 118
diet 7, 8, 9, 10, 17, 18, 19, 24, 32, 39, 40, 41, 42, 45, 48, 49, 51,
    56, 57, 60, 61, 63, 68, 69, 71, 72, 75, 77, 79, 80, 81, 84, 88,
    91, 92, 93, 96, 101, 103, 104, 105, 109
digestion 8, 69, 77, 94-95, 100, 104, 113, 114
dioxins 20
diuretic 13, 18, 53
diverticulosis 74

DMSO 98, 109
DNA 11, 23, 24, 40, 42, 78
dong quai 92
DPT vaccine 29

E

ear 7, 75-76, 111, 112, 117
ear candles 75
echinacea 40, 63, 66, 79, 97, 110, 113
elderberry 66, 97
ellagic acid 61
endometriosis 79-80
energy 7, 8, 9, 12, 13, 16, 18, 32, 34, 36, 40, 67, 70, 77, 78, 79,
      80, 81, 86, 89, 91, 92, 95, 96, 101, 103, 104, 109, 111
enzymes 8, 11, 23, 41, 44, 46, 52, 67, 69, 80, 94, 95, 113, 114
essential fatty acids 9, 45, 46, 49, 50, 58, 60, 67, 69, 70, 74, 78,
      80, 83, 87, 88, 92, 93, 99, 105, 108, 110, 115
essential oils 21, 59, 75, 97, 118
essiac 62, 73, 92, 117
evening primrose oil 50, 58, 61, 72, 92, 99, 105
exercise 15-16, 32-34, 52, 64, 69, 70, 71, 84, 88, 93, 94, 98, 103,
      108, 114
eye 21, 43, 48, 73, 74, 76, 77, 83, 118

F

5HTP 70, 99
fatigue 8, 13, 17, 18, 43, 49, 77, 79, 96, 99-111, 115, 123
fertility 12, 23, 96
fever 43, 65, 79, 96
feverfew 84
fibrin 115
fibroids 79
fibromyalgia 80
flatulence 10, 94, 95
flaxseed 45, 46, 50, 57, 60, 67, 69, 71, 74, 80, 83, 87, 88, 90, 99,
      105, 110

flu 30, 65, 66, 80, 96, 97, 102
fluoride 11, 12, 84, 96

G

GABA 70
gallbladder 81
garlic 53, 75, 79, 82, 86, 109
genetically engineered foods 24
ginger 66, 97, 102
ginkgo biloba 55, 93, 112
ginseng 72, 78, 87, 93
glutathione 40, 55, 76
gout 82
grapefruit seed extract 96, 105

H

hair 83
headache 11, 21, 83-84, 91, 96
heart 9, 10, 11, 13, 17, 18, 19, 21, 33, 34, 36, 37, 40, 54, 77, 78,
    83-87, 99, 103, 112, 115, 121, 122, 123
hemorrhoids 88
hepatitis 88
herpes 89
HGH 78, 80
hives 90
homeopathic 31
homocysteine 87
hormones 19, 20, 79-80, 91, 93, 99, 104
houseplants 16, 123

I

immunizations 26, 28
incontinence 94
infertility 96
influenza 96

insect bites 97-98
insomnia 17, 70, 91, 98-99
ipriflavone 105
irradiated food 23-24

J

joints 12, 44, 82

K

kava 70, 99
kelp 111

L

L-Carnitine 85
L-Glutamine 114
L-Lysine 64
L-Taurine 70
L-Tyrosine 70
learning disabilities 11
lecithin 50, 55, 119
licorice 42, 114
liver 21, 30, 42, 81, 88, 89, 112, 117
lungs 12, 15, 21, 46, 58, 107
lutein 76
lycopene 96
lymphatic system 56

M

magnesium 10, 11, 42, 46, 49, 51, 58, 59, 61, 68, 69, 70, 71, 72,
    73, 81, 84, 87, 91, 94, 98, 102, 104, 107, 112
magnet 109
melatonin 99
memory 11, 18-19, 22, 50, 55, 70

menopause 91, 99
mercury 50, 96
metal toxicity 100
methylcobalamin 106
microwave oven 21, 22, 23, 121
Miracle Oil 46, 58, 64, 97, 113, 118, 120
miscarriage 12, 91
MSG 18, 45, 83
MSM 42, 43, 44, 59, 66, 81, 83, 88, 89, 91, 100, 101, 110, 114
Multiple Sclerosis 101
music 34

N

nausea 17, 96, 102
nuts 9, 96, 119

O

obesity 8, 13, 28, 71, 88
olive leaf extract 51, 63, 66, 79, 87, 90, 105, 110, 113
organic 10, 14, 24, 89, 101
osteoporosis 11, 104
oxygen 8, 14, 15, 16, 17, 33, 56, 60, 62, 69, 78, 83, 84, 87, 95,
    107, 123

P

parasites 10, 66, 95, 105, 106, 118
Parkinson's Disease 18, 55, 106
pectin 86, 114
pH 17, 19, 95, 117
PMS 18, 58, 91
pneumonia 107
potassium 112
progesterone 80, 91
prostate 61, 62, 93, 94, 107, 108

protein 9, 41, 49, 50, 78, 81, 86, 87, 89, 92, 94, 103, 104, 119
psyllium husks 67
pycnogenol 73, 101, 106

Q

quercetin 83, 98

R

radiation 10, 21, 23, 24, 57, 63, 76
raw food 8, 9, 10, 41, 53, 74, 75, 80, 84, 92, 94, 104, 121
red clover 89
Rescue Remedy™ 50, 109
Ritalin 47

S

St. John's Wort 70
saliva 117
sciatica 108
seizure 17, 18, 28, 30, 98
selenium 40, 41, 50, 56, 60, 76, 86, 89, 96, 110, 113
shingles 109
Siberian ginseng 87, 93
SIDS 28, 29
silymarin 81, 89
sinusitis 109
skin 14, 19, 40, 43, 54, 59, 61, 62, 63, 70, 90, 91, 110, 115, 122
soft drinks 19, 57, 77, 94, 113
sore throat 58, 110, 118, 120
spirulina 41, 45, 50, 63, 78, 100, 103, 110
stress 32, 42, 49, 50, 64, 73, 77, 79, 83, 94, 95, 98, 100, 109,
    113, 114

T

tea 13, 17, 40, 51, 53, 54, 55, 57, 59, 62, 73, 75, 89, 92, 93, 97,

98, 102, 117, 120
tea tree oil 40, 51, 54, 63, 75, 89, 97, 98, 120
thirst 12-13
thoughts 34, 35, 36, 37, 38
thyroid 12, 77, 83, 98, 111
tinnitus 18, 111, 112
tooth decay 111, 113
toxins 8, 12, 13, 24, 66, 67, 88, 89, 95, 100, 114, 118, 123
Traditional Flower Remedies™ 44, 109
tumeric 45, 95

U

ulcers 113, 118
urine 52, 53, 82, 94, 104, 108

V

valerian 70, 81, 99
vanadyl sulfate 73
varicose veins 114
vitamin A 5, 41, 42, 43, 76, 112
vitamin C 5, 41, 42, 43, 44, 53, 56, 58, 59, 64, 65, 66, 71, 75
vitamin E 11, 41, 54, 57, 60, 71, 78, 80, 86, 88, 96, 99, 101, 107,
    109, 114

W

warts 115
water 7, 10, 11, 12, 13, 14, 16, 17, 18, 20, 25, 39, 40, 42, 43, 44,
    46, 51, 52, 53, 54, 55, 56, 58, 59, 61, 62, 63, 67, 68, 69, 73,
    74, 77, 80, 81, 82, 83, 84, 85, 86, 87, 88, 89, 95, 96, 100, 101,
    102, 103, 107, 108, 110, 111, 112, 113, 117, 118, 119, 120,
    121, 122
wheatgrass 80
wild yam 91, 92, 104
wormwood 106

Y

yohimbe 93

Z

zinc 40, 42, 54, 59, 60, 66, 71, 74, 83, 89, 90, 94, 96, 97, 107, 108, 113, 114

Notes